PLANT-BASED COOK'S GUIDE

A Recipe Book With a Large Assortment of Easy and Delicious Whole-Food Plant-Based Diet Recipes to Get You Started!

Botanika Green Way

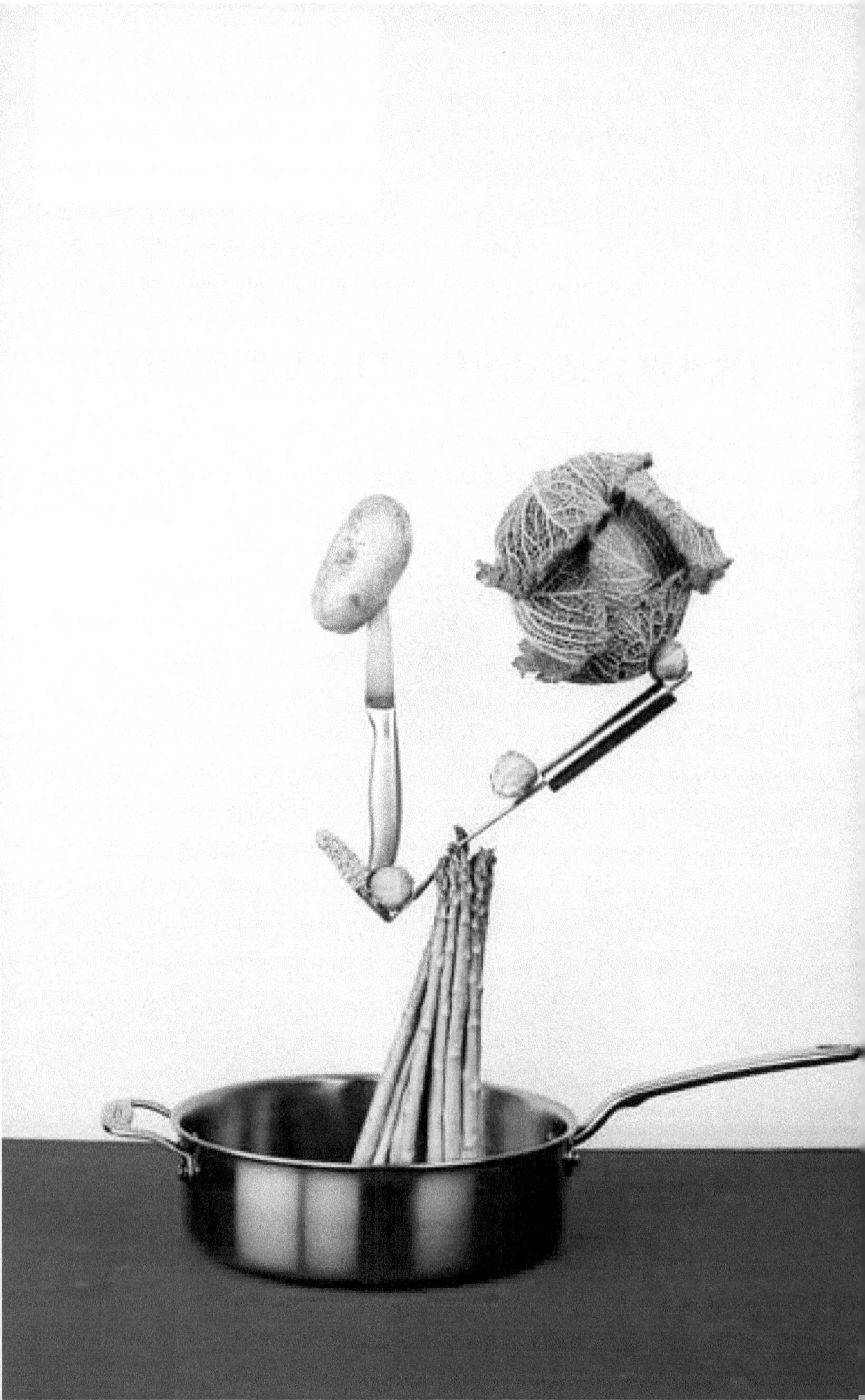

Table of Contents

INTRODUCTION

A plant-based diet is a diet based primarily on whole plant foods. Hence, it excludes animal-sourced foods, hydrogenated oils, refined sugars, and processed foods. A whole food plant-based diet does not consist solely of fruits and vegetables. It includes unprocessed or barely processed oils with healthy fats like extra-virgin olive oil, whole grains, legumes, seeds, and nuts, as well as herbs and spices.

What is the Plant-Based Diet?

The plant-based diet may seem similar to a vegetarian or vegan diet, but it is neither. It's not a diet but a healthy lifestyle. It uses food from plants, and it excludes processed foods like white rice and added sugars, which are allowed in vegan and vegetarian diets.

A plant-based diet is not a diet; it's a healthy way of life

The secret to a healthy diet is simpler than you ever thought! When following a plant-based dietary regimen, you should focus on plant-based foods and avoid animal-sourced food. Whether you are already following a vegan diet or are considering trying this lifestyle, this plant-based, budget-friendly food list makes your grocery shopping easy to manage.

- **VEGETABLES**

Try to include different types of vegetables in your diet from above-ground vegetables to root vegetables, which grow underground.

- **FRUITS**

Choose affordable fruits that are in season. Add frozen fruit to your grocery list since they are just as nutritious as fresh produce. They can be used in smoothies, toppings, compotes, or preserves. On the other hand, dried fruit generally contains a lot of antioxidants, especially polyphenols. It has been proven that eating dried fruits can prevent heart disease and some types of cancer.

- **NUTS & SEEDS**

Nuts and seeds offer different dietary benefits. They do not only ensure essential nutrients but are also offer a variety of flavors. This "ready to eat" food is a perfect snack with dried fruits and trail mix, essential vegan foods to stockpile for an emergency.

- **RICE & GRAINS**

Rice and grains are versatile and easy to incorporate into your diet. Leftovers reheat wonderfully and can be served at any time of the day, turning simple and inexpensive ingredients into a full-fledged meal. You can also make healthy nut butters such as tahini or peanut butter.

- **BEANS & LEGUMES**

Legumes and beans are highly affordable, and there's no end to the variety of tasty dishes you can cook with them. These humble but powerful foods are packed with vitamins, minerals, protein, and dietary fiber. In addition to being super-healthy and versatile, legumes pair very well with other proteins, vegetables, and grains.

- **HEALTHY FATS**

Don't underestimate the importance of quality fats in cooking. Coconut oil, olive oil, and avocado are always good to have on hand.

- **NON-DAIRY PRODUCTS**

Using a plant-based cheese or milk lends flavor, texture, and nutrition to your meals. You can find fantastic products on the market, and this book has many wonderful recipes for feta, vegan ricotta, and plant-based milk.

- **HERBS, SPICES & CONDIMENTS**

A handful of fresh herbs will add that little something extra to your soups, stews, dips, or casseroles. Condiments such as mustard, ketchup, vegan mayonnaise, and plant-based sauces can be used in salads, casseroles, and spreads. Choosing their distinctive flavors to complement vegetables, grains and legumes will help you to make the most of your vegan dishes. Herbs and spices are naturally plant-based, but play it safe and look for a label that says *Vegan-friendly*.

- **BAKING GOODS & CANNED GOODS**

These vegan essentials include all types of flour, baking powder, baking soda, and yeast. Further, cocoa powder, vegan chocolate, and sweeteners are good to have on hand. As for the healthy vegan sweeteners, opt for fresh or dried fruits, agave syrup, maple syrup, and stevia. When it comes to canned goods, stock your pantry with cooking essentials such as tomato, sauerkraut, pickles, low sodium chickpeas and beans, coconut milk, green chilies, pumpkin puree, tomato sauce, low sodium corn, and artichoke hearts. Thus, if you want to make sure you have nutritious, delicious, and quality meals for you and your family, having a vegan pantry is halfway there.

Why You Ought to Reduce Your Intake of Processed and Animal-Based Foods

You have heard over and over that processed food has adverse effects on your health. You might have also been told repeatedly to stay away from foods with lots of preservatives. However, you may have never heard any genuine or concrete facts about why these foods are unsafe. Consequently, let us properly dissect it to help you properly comprehend why you ought to stay away from these offenders.

- **They have massive habit-forming characteristics**

Humans have a predisposition toward being addicted to some specific foods; however, the reality is that the fault is not wholly ours.

Every one of the unhealthy treats we relish now and then triggers a dopamine release. This creates a pleasurable effect in our brain, but the excitement is usually short-lived. The discharged dopamine gradually causes an attachment, and this is the reason some people consistently go back to eat certain unhealthy foods even when they know they're unhealthy and unnecessary. You can get rid of this by avoiding the temptation completely.

- **They are sugar-laden and heavy in glucose-fructose syrup**

Animal-based and processed foods are laden with refined sugars and glucose-fructose syrup, which has almost no nutritional value. An ever-increasing number of studies are affirming what several people presumed from the start: that genetically modified foods bring about inflammatory bowel disease, which consequently makes it increasingly difficult for the body to assimilate essential nutrients. The disadvantages that result from your body being unable to assimilate essential nutrients from consumed foods rightly cannot be overemphasized.

Processed and animal-based food products contain plenteous amounts of refined carbohydrates. Indeed, your body requires carbohydrates to give it energy to function.

In any case, refining carbs dispenses with the fundamental supplements in the way that refining entire grains disposes of the whole grain part. What remains in the wake of refining is what's considered empty carbs or empty calories. These can negatively affect the metabolic system in your body by sharply increasing your blood sugar and insulin levels.

- **They contain lots of synthetic ingredients**

When your body takes in non-natural ingredients, it regards them as foreign substance sand a health threat. It isn't accustomed to identifying synthetic compounds like sucralose or synthesized sugars. Hence, in defense of your health against this foreign "aggressor," your body does what it's programmed to do to safeguard your health: It sets off an immune reaction to tackle this "enemy" compound, which indirectly weakens your body's general disease alertness, making you susceptible to illnesses. The energy expended by your body in triggering your immune system could be better utilized somewhere else.

- **They contain constituent elements that set off a sensation in your body**

A part of processed and animal-based foods contains compounds like glucose-fructose syrup, monosodium glutamate, and specific food dyes that can trigger some addictions. They teach your body to receive a benefit whenever you consume them. Monosodium glutamate, for example, is added to many store-bought baked foods. This additive slowly conditions your palate to relish and crave the taste.

- **This reward-centric arrangement makes you crave it increasingly, which ends up exposing you to the danger of over-consuming calories**

For animal protein, usually, the expression “subpar” is used to allude to plant proteins since they generally have lower levels of essential amino acids as against animal-sourced protein. Nevertheless, what the vast majority don’t know is that large amounts of essential amino acids can prove detrimental to your health. Let me break it down further for you.

- **Animal-sourced protein has no fiber**

In their pursuit to consume animal protein, the vast majority wind up dislodging the plant protein that was previously available in their body. Replacing the plant proteins with its animal variant is harmful because, in contrast to plant protein, animal proteins typically are deficient in fiber, phyto-nutrients, and antioxidant properties. Fiber insufficiency is a regular feature across various regions and societies on the planet. In America, for example, according to the National Academy of Medicine, the typical adult takes in roughly 15 grams of dietary fiber daily rather than the recommended daily quantity of 25 to 30 grams. A deficiency in dietary fiber often leads to a heightened risk of breast and colorectal cancers, in addition to constipation, inflammatory bowel disease, and cardiovascular disease.

- **Animal protein brings about an upsurge in phosphorus levels in the body**

Animal protein has significant levels of phosphorus. Our bodies stabilize these plenteous amounts of phosphorus by producing and discharging a hormone known as fibroblast growth factor 23 (FGF23). Studies have shown that this hormone is dangerous to our veins. FGF23 also causes asymmetrical expansion of heart muscles—a determinant for congestive heart failure and even mortality in some advanced cases.

Having discussed the many problems associated with animal protein, it becomes more apt to replace its "high quality" perception with the tag "highly hazardous." In contrast to caffeine, which has a withdrawal effect if it's discontinued abruptly, you can stop taking processed and animal-based foods right away without any withdrawals. Possibly the only thing that you'll give up is the ease of some meals taking little tono time to prepare.

Health Benefits of the Plant-Based Diet

Plant-based eating is one of the healthiest diets in the world. It should include plenty of fresh products, whole grains, legumes, and healthy fats such as seeds and nuts, which are rich in antioxidants, minerals, vitamins, and dietary fiber.

Scientific research has shown that higher use of plant-based foods is connected to a lower risk of death from conditions such as cardiovascular disease, diabetes, hypertension, and obesity. Vegan eating relies heavily on healthy staples, avoiding animal products. Animal products contain much more fat than plant-based foods; it's not a shocker that studies have shown that meat-eaters have nine times the obesity rate of vegans.

This leads us to the next point, one of the greatest benefits of the vegan diet: weight loss. While many people choose to live a vegan life for ethical reasons, the diet itself can help you achieve your weight loss goals. If you're struggling to shift pounds, you may want to consider trying a plant-based diet. How exactly? As a vegan, you will reduce the number of high-calorie foods such as full-fat dairy products, fatty fish, pork, and other cholesterol-containing foods such as eggs. Try replacing such foods with high-fiber and protein-rich alternatives that will keep you fuller longer. The key is focusing on nutrient-dense, clean and natural foods and avoiding empty calories such as sugar, saturated fats, and highly processed foods. Here are a few tricks that help me maintain my weight on the vegan diet. I eat vegetables as a main course; I consume good fats in moderation (good fats such as olive oil do not make you fat); I exercise regularly and cook at home. Plant foods are an excellent source of many nutrients that boost the body's metabolism in many ways. They are easy to digest thanks to their rich content of antioxidants.

- **Reduced Risk of Heart Diseases**

Processed and animal foods are responsible for much heart disease. A whole foods plant-based diet is better at nourishing the body with essential nutrients while improving the heart's function to produce and transport blood to and from the various body parts.

- **Prevents and Heals Diabetes**

Plant-based foods are excellent at reducing high blood sugar. Many studies comparing a vegetarian and vegan diet to a regular meat-filled diet proved that dieting with more plant foods reduced the risk of diabetes by 50 percent.

- **Improved Cognitive Incline**

Fruits and vegetables are excellent for cleansing and boosting metabolism. They release high numbers of plant compounds and antioxidants that slow or prevent cognitive decline. On a plant-based diet, the brain is boosted with sustainable energy, promoting sharp memory, language, thinking, and judgment abilities.

- **Quick Weight Loss**

A high animal food diet is known to drive weight gain. Switching to a plant-based diet helps the body shed fat walls easily, which quickly drives weight loss.

BREAKFAST

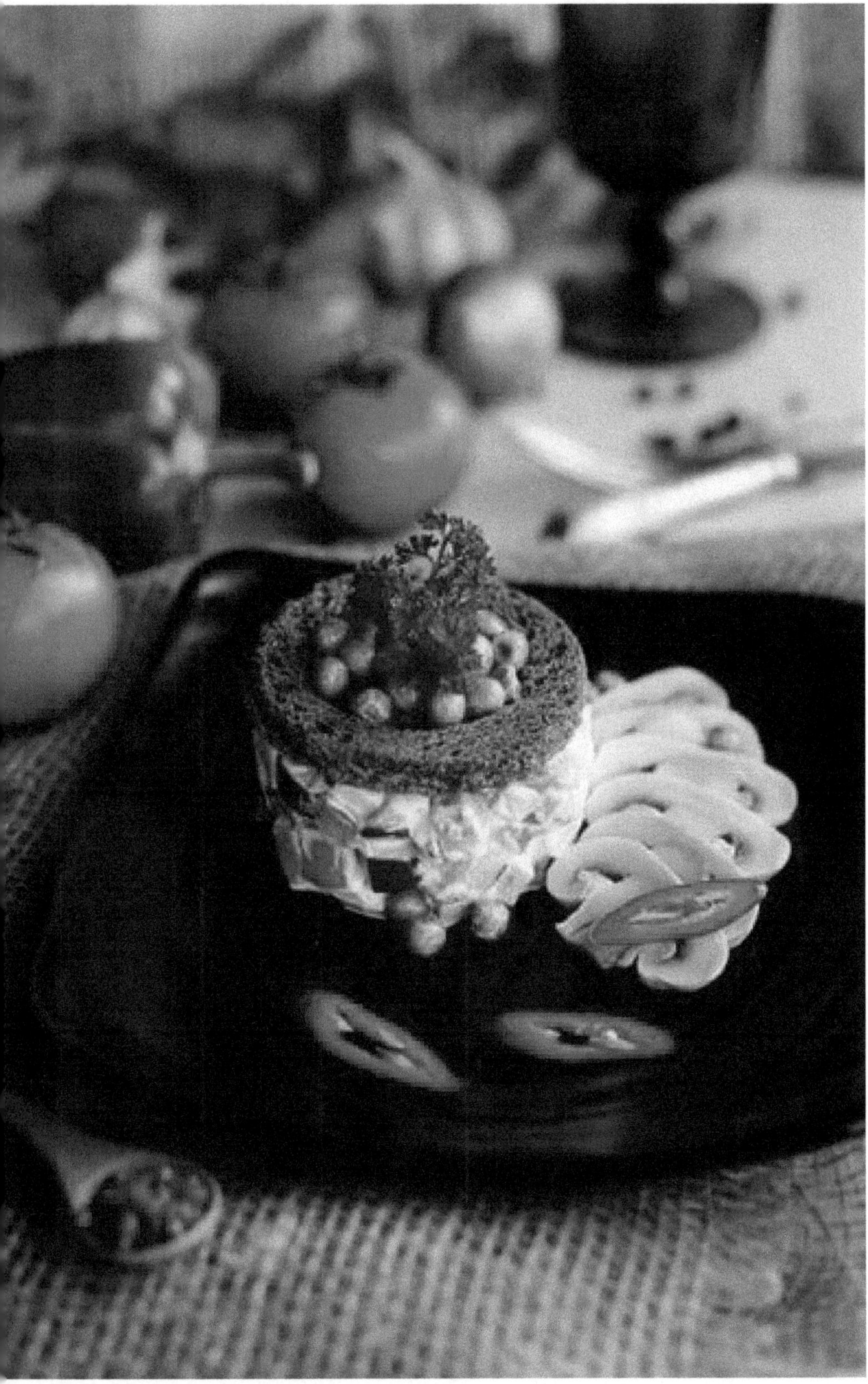

Coconut Blueberry Muffins

8 Servings

Preparation Time: 30 minutes

Ingredients

- 1 tbsp Coconut oil melted
- 1 tsp Almond extract
- 1 tsp Apple cider vinegar
- 1 ½ cups Whole-wheat flour
- ½ cup pure Date sugar
- 2 tsps Baking soda
- A pinch of Salt
- 1 cup Blueberries
- 1 cup quick-cooking Oats
- 1 cup boiling Water
- ½ cup almond Milk
- ¼ cup ground Flaxseed

Directions

- Preheat oven to 400°F.

- In a bowl, stir in the oats with boiling water until they are softened.

- Add in the coconut oil, milk, flaxseed, almond extract, and vinegar.

- Add in the flour, sugar, baking soda, and salt. Gently stir in blueberries.
- Divide the batter between a greased with coconut oil muffin tin. Bake for 20 minutes until lightly brown.
- Allow cooling for 10 minutes. Using a spatula, run the sides of the muffins to take out. Serve.

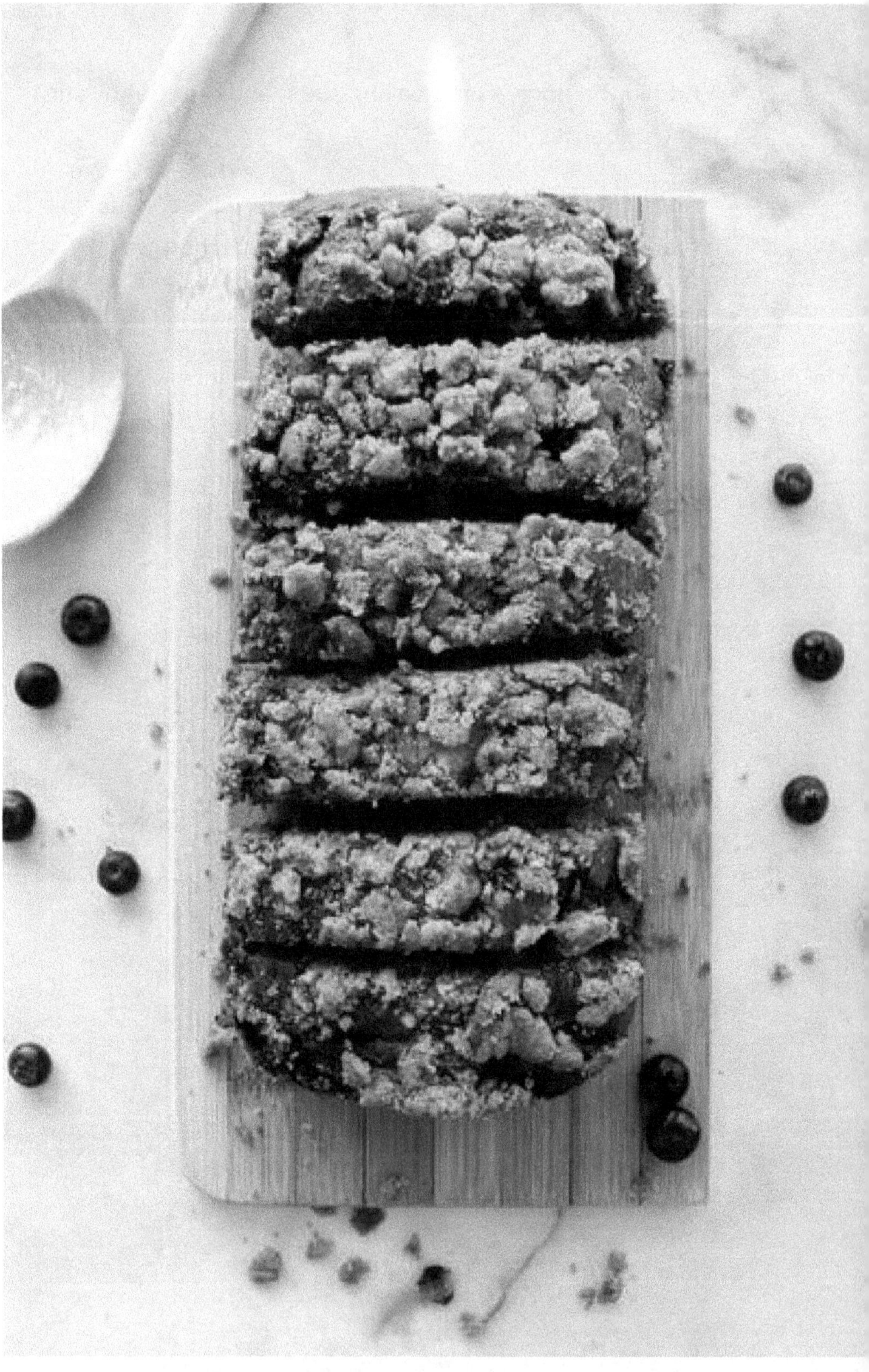

Scrambled Tofu with Swiss Chard

7 Servings

Preparation Time: 35 minutes

Ingredients

- 1 (14-oz) package Tofu, crumbled
- 1 Celery stalk, chopped
- 2 large Carrots, chopped
- 1 tsp Chili powder
- ½ tsp ground Cumin
- ½ tsp ground Turmeric
- Salt and Black pepper to taste
- 5 cups Swiss chard
- 2 tsps Olive oil
- 1 Onion, chopped
- 3 cloves minced garlic

Directions

- Heat the oil in a pan over medium heat.
- Add in the onion, garlic, celery, and carrots. Sauté for 5 minutes.
- Stir in tofu, chili powder, cumin, turmeric, salt, and pepper, cook for 7-8 minutes more.
- Mix in the Swiss chard and cook until wilted, about 3 minutes. Allow cooling and seal and serve.

Tangerine Banana Toast

6 Servings

Preparation Time: 25 minutes

Ingredients

- 3 Bananas
- 1 tsp ground Cinnamon
- ¼ tsp grated Nutmeg
- 4 slices Bread
- 1 tbsp Olive oil
- 1 cup Almond milk
- 1 Zest and juice of tangerine

Directions and

- Blend the bananas, almond milk, tangerine juice, tangerine zest, cinnamon, and nutmeg until smooth in a blender.

- Spread into a baking dish. Submerge the bread slices in the mixture for 3-4 minutes.

- Heat the oil in a pan over medium heat. Fry the bread for 5 minutes until golden brown. Serve hot.

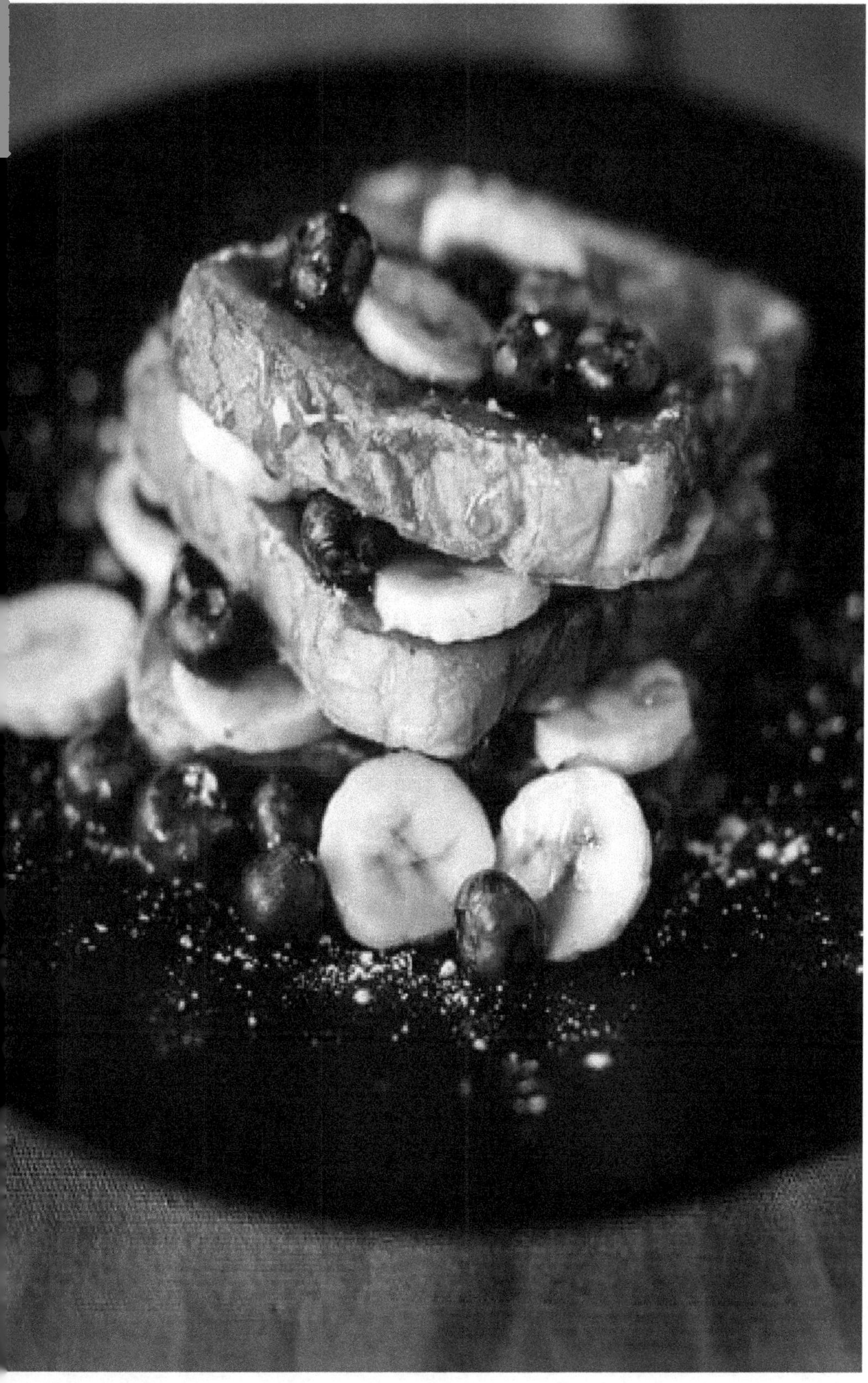

Energy Chia-Peach Smoothie

4 Servings

Preparation Time: 5 minutes

Ingredients

- 2 Bananas, sliced
- 2 scoops plant-based Protein powder
- 2 tbsps Chia seeds
- 2 Cucumbers, chopped
- 2 Peaches, chopped
- 2 cups Almond milk

Directions

- Purée the banana, peach, almond milk, protein powder, chia seeds, and cucumber for 50 seconds until smooth in a blender.

- Serve immediately in glasses.

Mango Rice Pudding

6 Servings

Preparation Time: 30 minutes

Ingredients

- 1 cup Brown rice
- 2 tsps Pumpkin pie spice
- 1 Mango, chopped
- 2 tbsps Chopped walnuts
- 1 ½ cups Non-dairy milk
- 3 tbsps Pure date sugar

Directions

- In a pot over medium heat, add in the rice, 2 cups water, milk, sugar, and pumpkin pie spice.

- Bring to a boil, lower the heat and simmer for 18-20 minutes until the rice is soft and the liquid is absorbed.

- Put in the mango and stir to combine. Top with walnuts to serve.

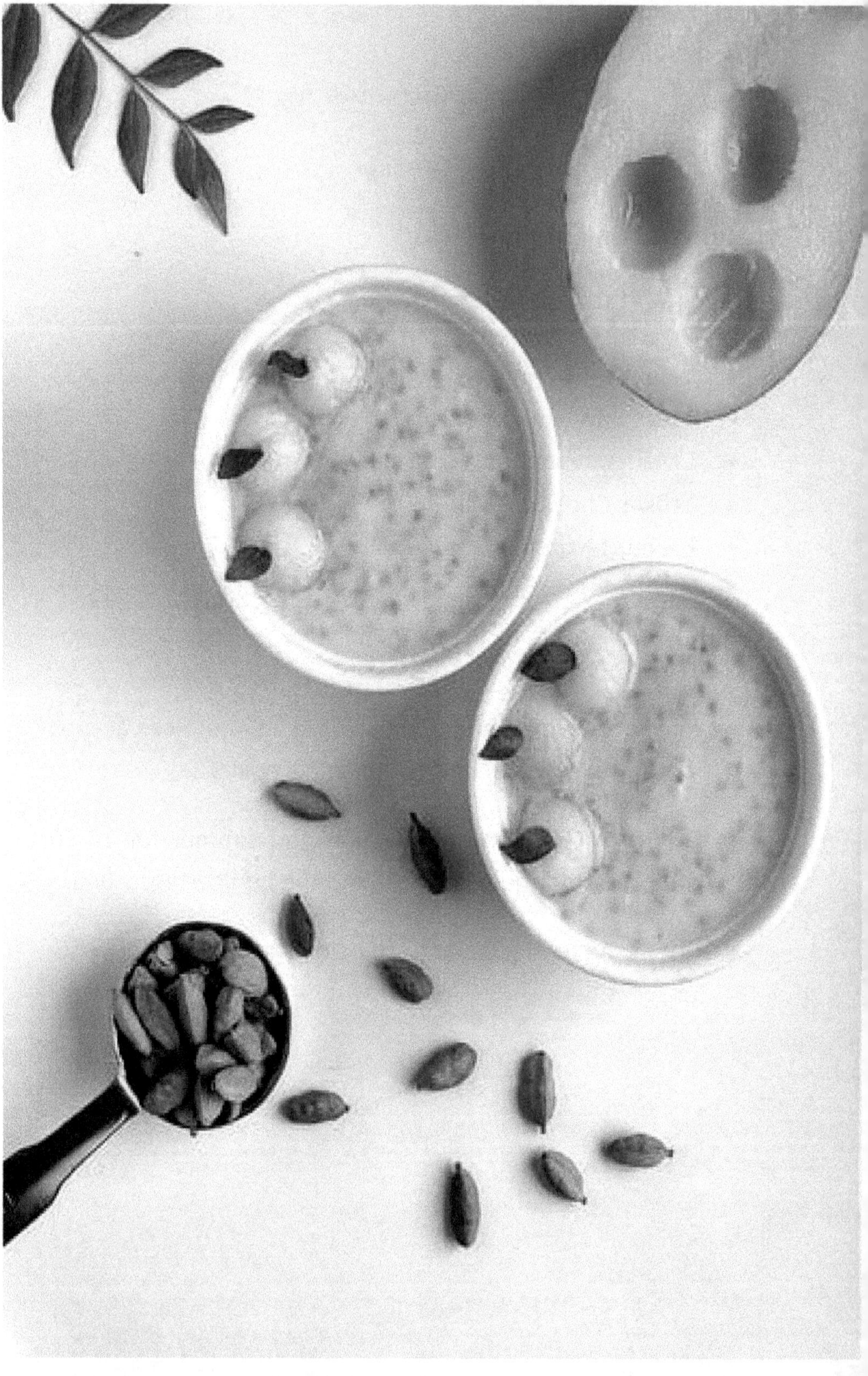

Tropical Smoothie Bowl

6 Servings

Preparation Time: 10 minutes

Ingredients

- 6 Bananas, sliced
- 3 cups fresh Raspberries
- ½ cup slivered Almonds
- 4 cups plant-based Milk
- 1 cup Papaya
- 1 cup Baked granola, crushed

Directions

- Put bananas, raspberries, and milk in a blender and blend until smooth.

- Transfer to a bowl and stir in granola. Top with almonds and serve.

Coconut Fruit Smoothie

5 Servings

Preparation Time: 5 minutes

Ingredients

- 1 cup Strawberries
- ½ cup Coconut milk
- 1 cup Water
- 1 tsp Goji berries
- 2 tbsps Fresh mint, chopped
- 1 cup chopped Watermelon
- 1 cup Cranberries
- 1 tbsp Chia seeds

Directions

- In a blender, put the strawberries, watermelon, cranberries, chia seeds, coconut milk, water, goji berries, and mint.

- Blend until smooth, adding more water or milk if needed. Divide between 5 glasses and serve.

DRINKS

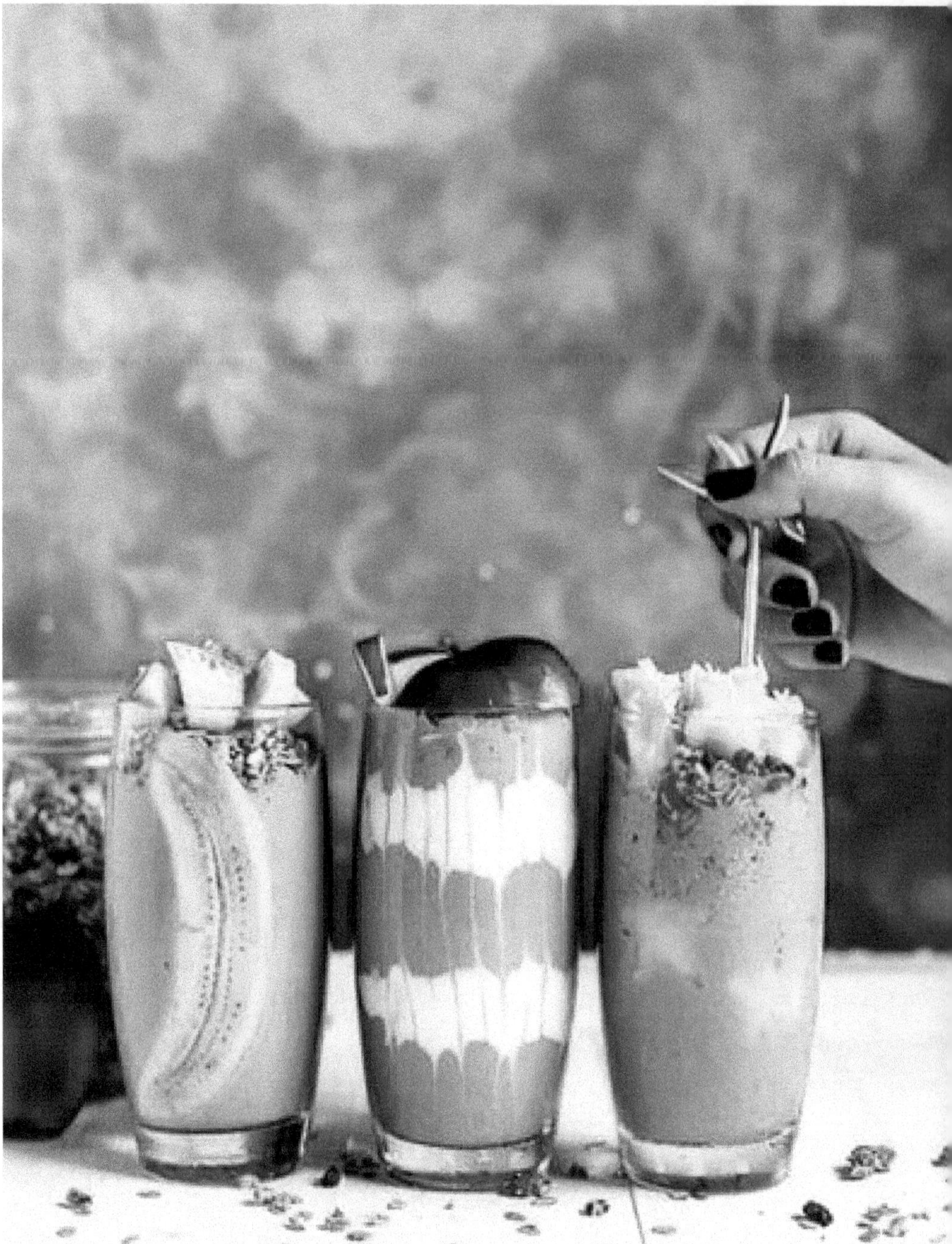

Strawberry Beet Smoothie

2 Servings

Preparation Time: 5 minutes

Ingredients

- 1 red beet, trimmed, peeled, and chopped into cubes
- 1 cup strawberries, quartered
- 1 ripe banana
- ½ cup strawberry yogurt
- 1 Tbsp honey
- 1 Tbsp water
- Milk, to taste

Directions

- Sprinkle the beet cubes with water, place them on aluminum foil, and put them in the oven (preheated to 204°C). Bake for 40 minutes.
- Let the baked beet cool.
- Combine all the smoothie ingredients.
- Enjoy your fantastic drink.

Creamy Avocado Drink

4 Servings

Preparation Time: 55 minutes

Ingredients

- 4 large ripe avocados, halved and pitted
- 4 tbsps swerve sugar
- ¼ cup cold almond milk
- 1 tsp vanilla extract
- 1 tbsp cold heavy cream

Directions

- In a blender, add the avocado pulp, swerve sugar, almond milk, vanilla extract, and heavy cream. Process until smooth.
- Pour the mixture into 2 tall serving glasses, garnish with strawberries, and serve immediately.

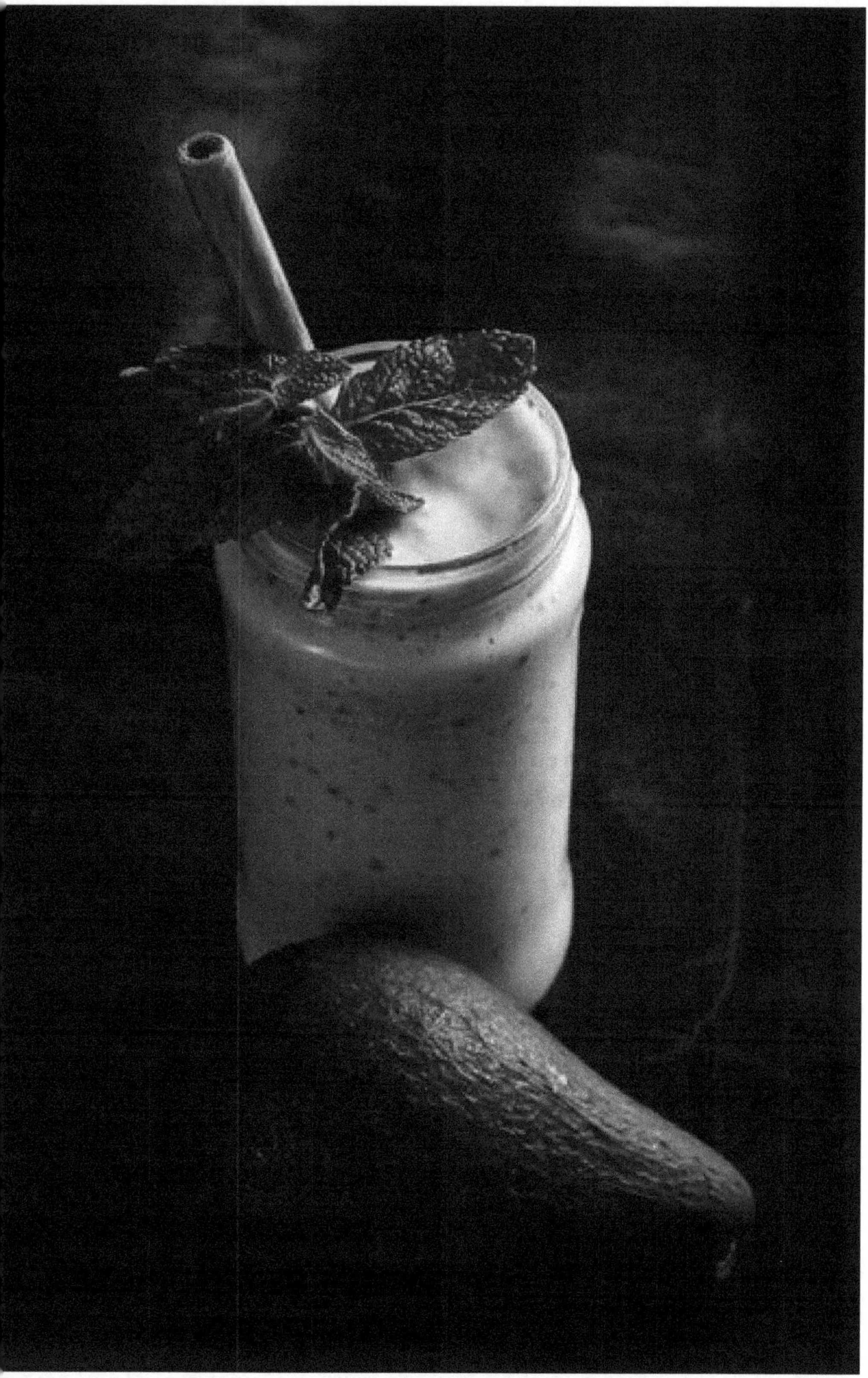

Chocolatey Banana Shake

2 Servings

Preparation Time: 10 minutes

Ingredients

- 2 medium frozen bananas, peeled
- 4 dates, pitted
- 4 tablespoons peanut butter
- 4 tablespoons rolled oats
- 2 tablespoons cacao powder
- 2 tablespoons chia seeds
- 2 cups unsweetened soymilk

Directions

- Place all the ingredients in a high-speed blender and pulse until creamy.
- Pour into two glasses and serve immediately.

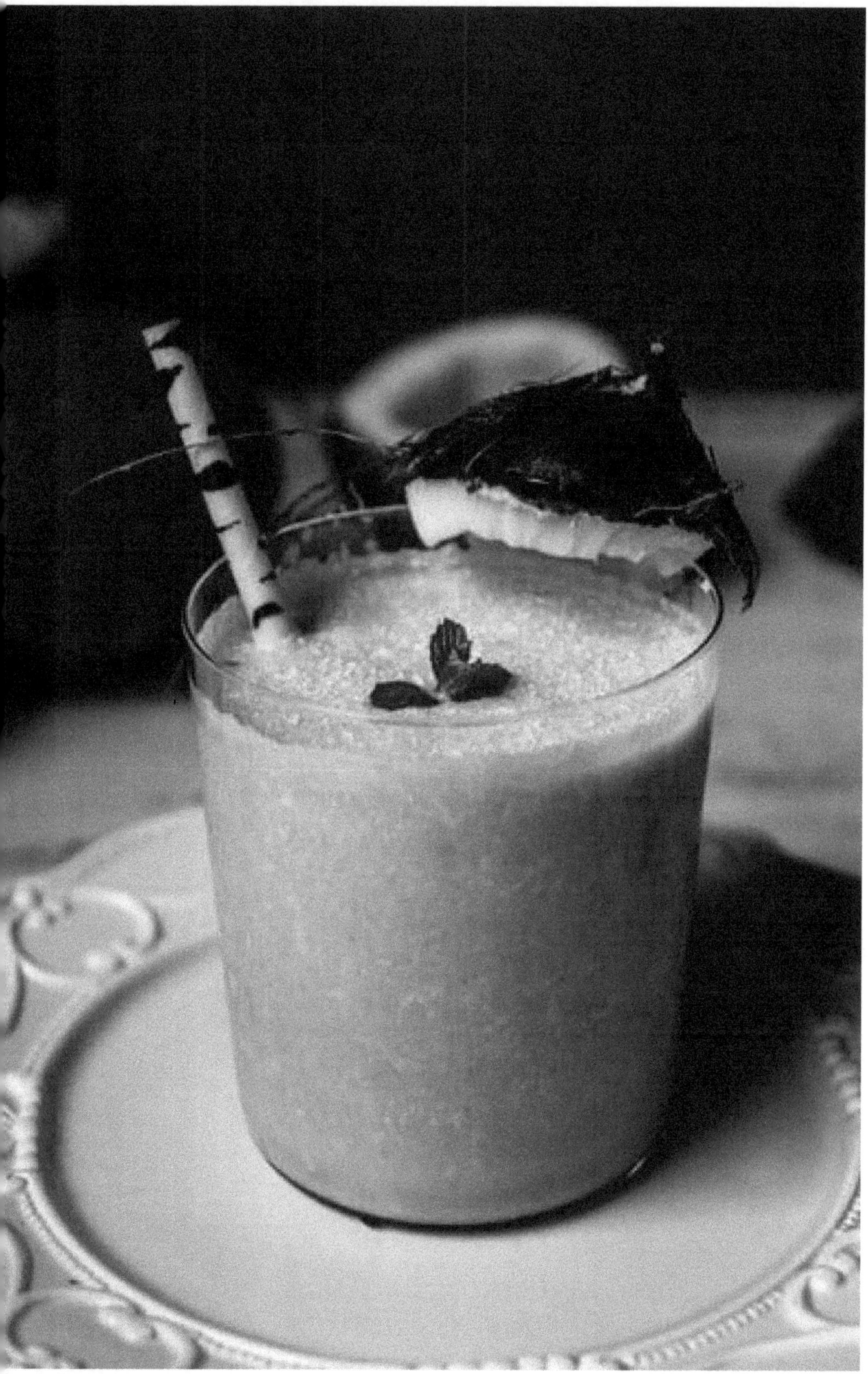

Fruity Tofu Smoothie

2 Servings

Preparation Time: 10 minutes

Ingredients

- 12 ounces silken tofu, pressed and drained
- 2 medium bananas, peeled
- 1½ cups fresh blueberries
- 1 tablespoon maple syrup
- 1½ cups unsweetened soymilk
- ¼ cup of ice cubes

Directions

- Place all the ingredients in a high-speed blender and pulse until creamy.
- Pour into two glasses and serve immediately.

LUNCH

Hot Lentil Tacos with Guacamole

6 Servings

Preparation Time: 35 minutes

Ingredients

- ½ cup red Lentils, rinsed and drained
- 1 tbsp minced fresh Parsley
- 2 tsps hot powder
- Salt to taste
- 4 corn tortillas, warmed and halved
- Shredded romaine lettuce
- Guacamole
- 2 tbsps olive oil
- ½ cup minced onion
- 1 potato, peeled and shredded
- ½ cup roasted cashews
- ¼ cup chickpea flour

Directions

- Place the lentils in a pot and cover them with cold water. Bring to a boil and simmer for 15-20 minutes. Heat the oil in a pan over medium heat.

- Place in onion and potato and cook for 5 minutes. Set aside.

- In a blender, mince cashews, add in cooked lentils and onion mixture. Pulse to blend. Transfer to a bowl and stir in flour, parsley, hot powder, and salt.
- Mix to combine. Mold 8 patties out of the mixture.
- Heat the remaining oil in a skillet over medium heat. Brown the patties for 10 minutes on both sides. To assemble, put one cake in each tortilla, top with shredded lettuce and guacamole.

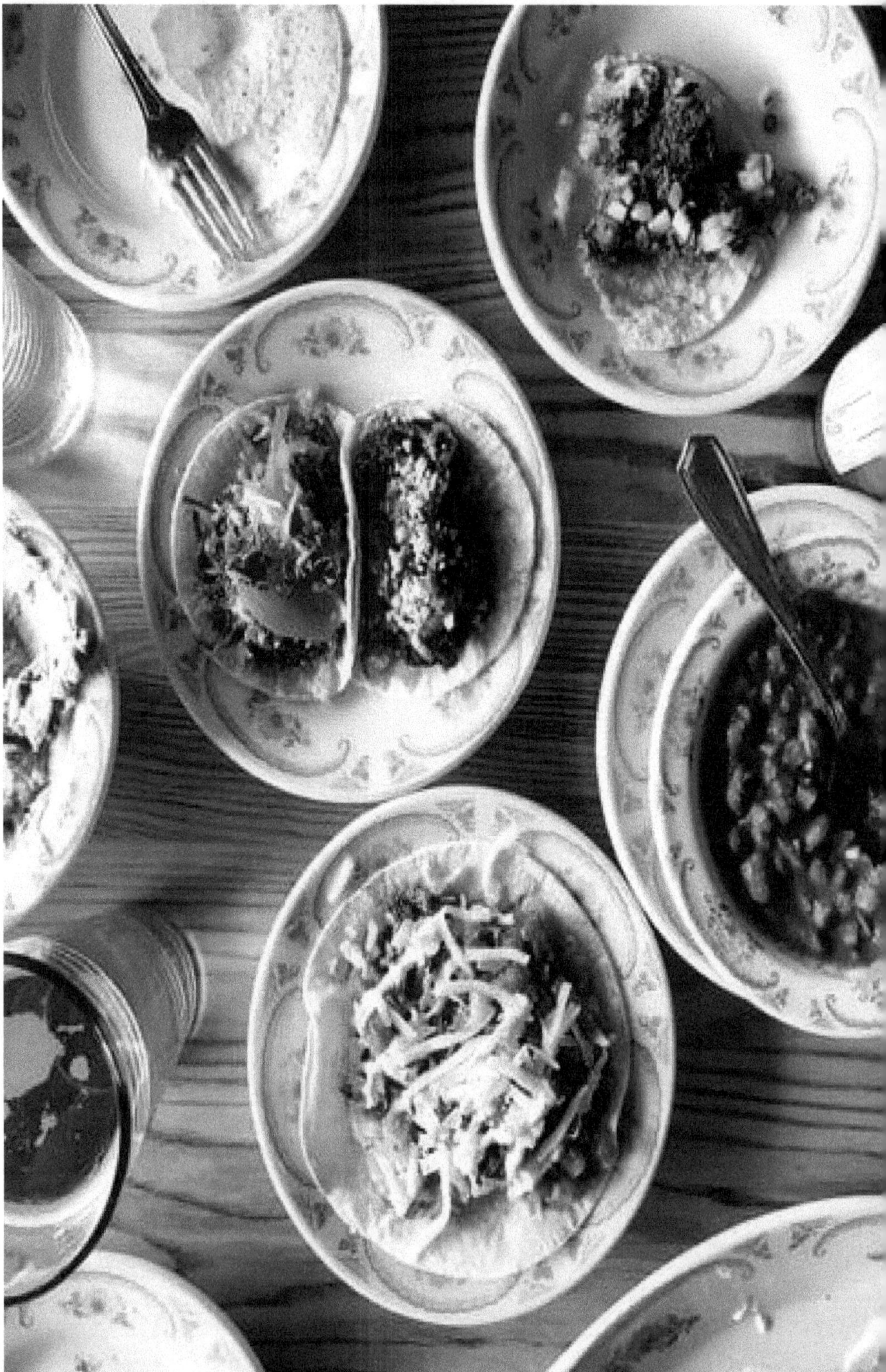

Curried Indian Rolls

6 Servings

Preparation Time: 15 minutes

Ingredients

- 3 tbsps tahini
- Zest and juice of 1 lime
- 1 tbsp curry powder
- 1 cup diced peaches
- 1 red bell pepper, diced small
- ½ cup fresh cilantro, chopped
- 4 large whole-grain wraps
- 2 cups shredded Iceberg lettuce
- Sea salt to taste
- 3 tbsps water
- 1 (14-oz) can chickpeas, drained

Directions

- In a bowl, beat tahini, lime zest, lime juice, curry powder, 3-4 tbsps of water, and salt until creamy.
- In another bowl, combine the chickpeas, peaches, bell pepper, cilantro, and tahini dressing.
- Divide the mixture between the wraps and top with lettuce.
- Roll up and serve.

Dijon Faro & Walnut Salad

6 Servings

Preparation Time: 50 minutes

Ingredients

- 1 cup faro
- ¼ cup olive oil
- ½ tsp dried oregano
- Salt and black pepper to taste
- ½ cup chopped red bell peppers
- 1/3 cup chopped toasted walnuts
- 2 tbsps minced fresh parsley
- 1 red onion, sliced
- 1 garlic clove, minced
- 2 tbsps white wine vinegar
- 1 tbsp Dijon mustard

Directions

- Cook faro in salted water for 25 minutes.
- Drain and set aside to cool.
- In a bowl, put the onion, garlic, vinegar, mustard, oil, oregano, salt, and pepper. Mix to combine.
- To the cooled faro, add bell peppers, walnuts, and parsley; stir
- Transfer to a serving plate, drizzle with the onion mixture, and serve.

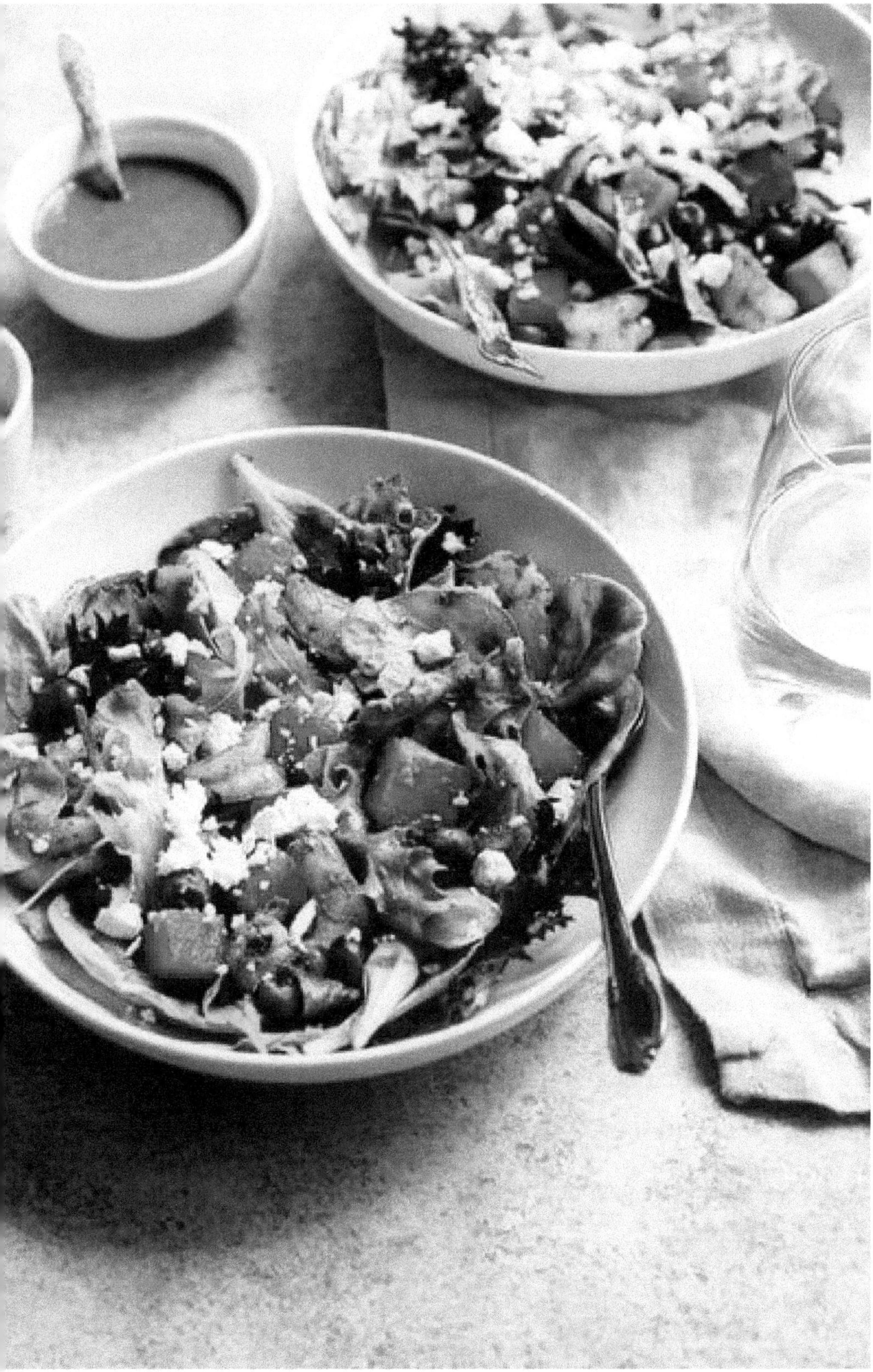

Awesome Barley Jambalaya

6 Servings

Preparation Time: 25 minutes

Ingredients

- 2 tbsps Olive oil
- 2 (15.5-oz) cans kidney beans
- 1 (14.5-oz) can diced Tomatoes
- 1 tsp dried Rosemary
- 2 ½ cups vegetable broth
- 1 tbsp chopped fresh Parsley
- Sriracha sauce
- 1 Onion, chopped
- 2 Celery stalks, chopped
- 1 Green bell peppers, chopped
- 2 Garlic cloves, minced
- 1 cup pearl Barley

Directions

- Heat the oil in a pot over medium heat.
- Place in onion, celery, bell pepper, and garlic. Sauté for 5 minutes.
- Add in barley, beans, tomatoes, rosemary, salt, and pepper.

- Stir in broth and simmer for 15 minutes.
- Top with parsley and drizzle with sriracha sauce to serve.

Baked Mustard Beans

6 Servings

Preparation Time: 25 minutes

Ingredients

- 2 tbsps Olive oil
- ½ cup pure Date syrup
- 1 ½ tsps dry Mustard
- ¼ tsp ground Cayenne pepper
- Salt and black pepper to taste
- 2 (15.5-oz) cans Great Northern beans
- 1 Onion, minced
- 2 Garlic cloves, minced
- 1 (14.5-oz) can crushed tomatoes

Directions

- Preheat oven to 350 F.
- Heat the oil in a pot over medium heat.
- Place in onion and garlic and sauté for 3 minutes.
- Add in tomatoes, date syrup, mustard, cayenne pepper, salt, and pepper. Cook for 5 minutes.
- Pour the beans into a baking dish and stir in the sauce to coat.
- Bake for 10 minutes. Serve warm.

Hot Bean Salad

6 Servings

Preparation Time: 45 minutes

Ingredients

- 1 cup pinto Beans, soaked overnight
- 1/3 cup chopped green Onions
- 1 tbsp chopped fresh Parsley
- 2 tbsps Olive oil
- 2 tbsps Balsamic vinegar
- Salt and black pepper to taste
- 4 Tomatoes, halved and sliced
- 2 celery stalks, sliced
- 2 hot chilies, seeded and minced

Directions

- Cook pinto beans in salted water for 40 minutes. Drain and remove to a bowl.
- Let cool for a few minutes.
- Stir in tomatoes, celery, chilies, and green onions.
- In another bowl, mix olive oil, vinegar, salt, and pepper.
- Add the dressing to the bean bowl and toss to coat.
- Transfer to a serving plate. Top with parsley and serve.

Rice, Lentil & Spinach Pilaf

6 Servings

Preparation Time: 25 minutes

Ingredients

- ½ cup Wild rice
- 1 tsp dried Thyme
- Salt and black pepper to taste
- 3 cups fresh baby Spinach
- 1 (15.5-oz) can Lentils, drained
- 1 (14.5-oz) can diced Tomatoes

Directions

- In a pot over medium heat, bring the rice and 1 ½ cups of salted water to a boil.
- Reduce the heat, cover, and simmer for 20 minutes.
- Add in lentils, tomatoes, thyme, salt, and pepper.
- Stir and cook until heated through.
- Mix in the spinach, cook for 2 minutes until the spinach wilts. Serve warm.

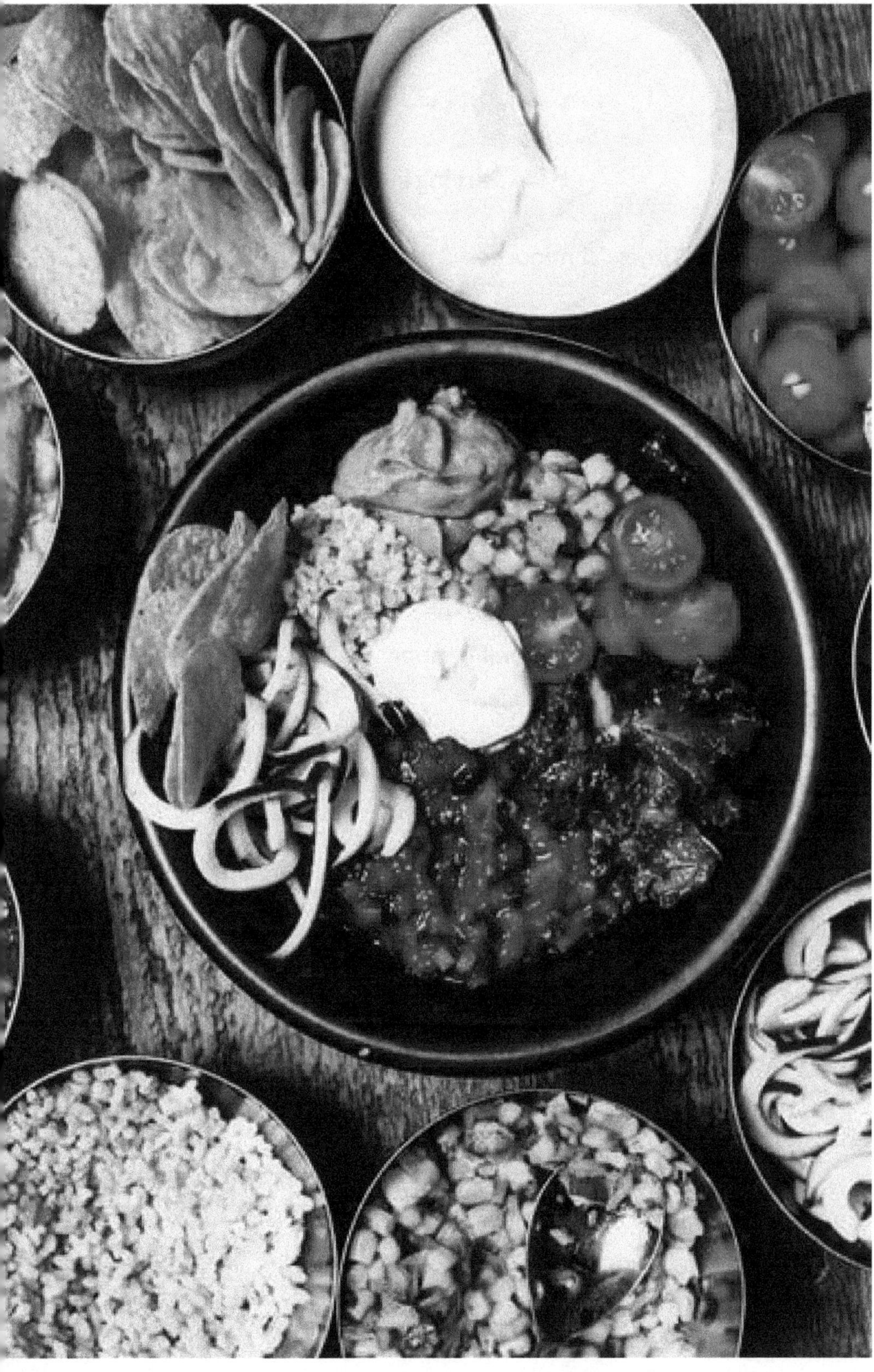

Parsley Bean & Olives Salad

6 Servings

Preparation Time: 15 minutes

Ingredients

- 1 cup Green olives, pitted and sliced
- ¼ cup chopped fresh Parsley
- Salt and Black pepper to taste
- 2 tbsps fresh Lime juice
- ¼ cup olive oil
- 2 (15.5-oz) cans black beans
- ½ cup chopped red bell pepper
- ¼ cup red Onions, sliced
- 2 Garlic cloves, crushed

Directions

- Combine the olives, beans, bell pepper, and onion in a bowl. Set aside.
- In a blender, put garlic, lime juice, 2 tbsps water, olive oil, parsley, salt, and pepper.
- Pulse until blended.
- Add to the salad bowl and mix to combine Serve immediately.

Cucumber & Carrot Pizza with Pesto

6 Servings

Preparation Time: 30 minutes

Ingredients

- 1 Prebaked pizza crust
- 1 Carrot, grated
- 1 red Onion, sliced
- 1 Cucumber, sliced
- ½ cup vegan pesto
- 1 Tomato, sliced

Directions

- Preheat oven to 390 F.
- Spread half of the pesto over the pizza crust and top with tomato slices.
- Combine the grated carrot with salt, toss to coat.
- Put the carrot over the tomato and top with onion.
- Transfer to a baking tray and put it in the oven.
- Bake for 15-20 minutes until golden. Serve topped with cucumber slices.

SOUPS & SALADS

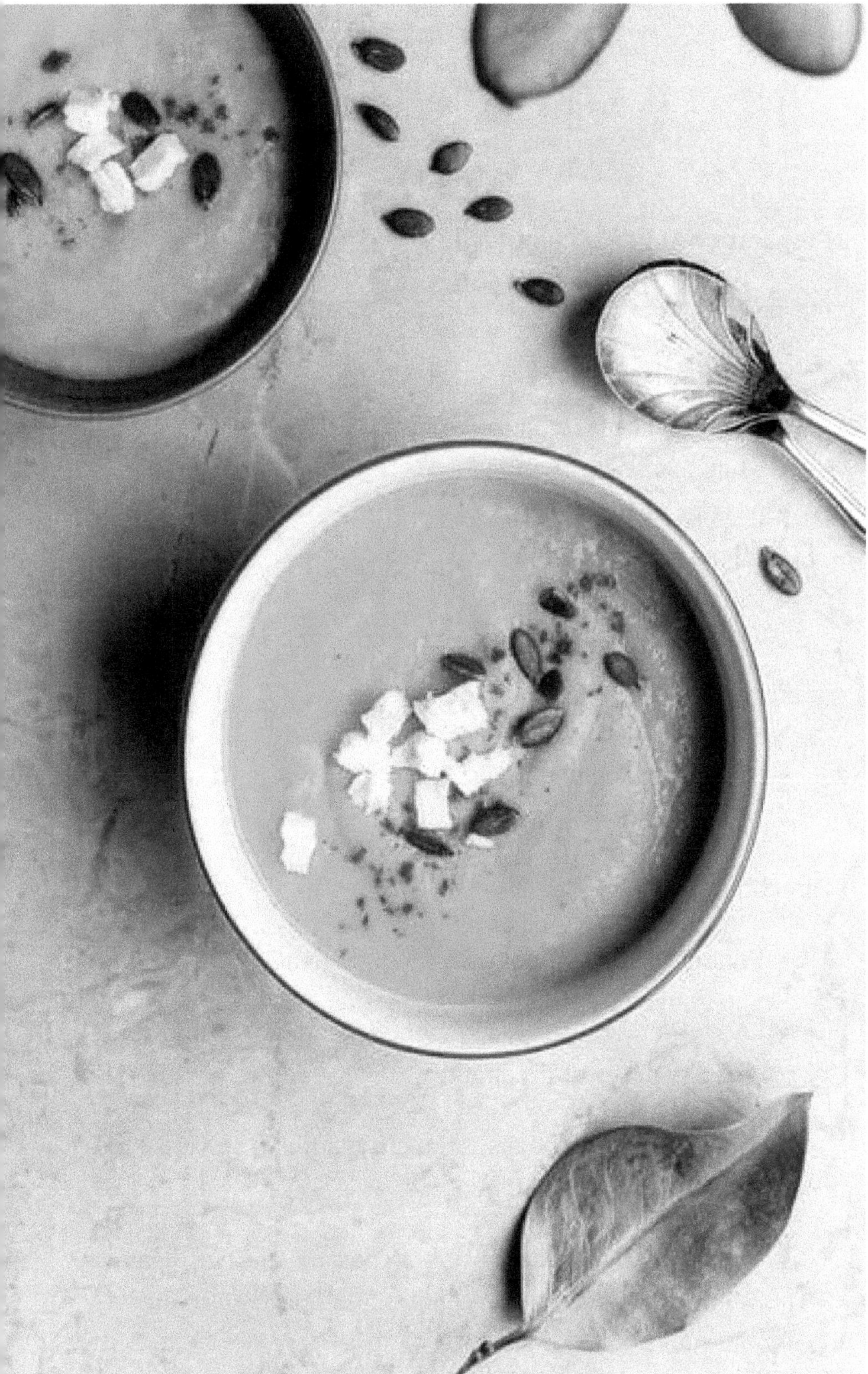

Easy Garbanzo Soup

6 Servings

Preparation Time: 25 minutes

Ingredients

- 2 tbsps Olive oil
- 1 (15-oz) can Garbanzo beans
- 1 cup Spinach, chopped
- 4 cups Vegetable stock
- ¼ tsp ground Cumin
- Sea salt to taste
- ¼ cup chopped Cilantro
- 1 Onion, chopped
- 1 Green bell pepper, diced
- 1 Carrot, peeled and diced
- 4 Garlic cloves, minced

Directions

- Warm the oil in a pot over medium heat.
- Add in onion, garlic, bell pepper, and carrot and sauté for 5 minutes until tender.
- Stir in garbanzo beans, spinach, vegetable stock, cumin, and salt. Cook for 10 minutes.
- Mash the garbanzo using a potato masher, leaving some chunks. Top with cilantro and serve.

Noodle Soup

8 Servings

Preparation Time: 30 minutes

Ingredients

- 2 tbsps Olive oil
- 1 (28-oz) can crushed Tomatoes
- 1 cup Chana dal, rinsed and drained
- 1 tsp dried Thyme
- 6 cups vegetable broth
- 4 oz Soba noodles, broken into thirds
- 1 Onion, chopped
- 1 Carrot, sliced
- 2 Garlic cloves, minced

Directions

- Heat the oil in a pot over medium heat.
- Add in onion, carrot, and garlic and sauté for 5 minutes.
- Add in tomatoes, chana dal, thyme, and broth.
- Bring to a boil, then lower the heat and season with salt and pepper.
- Simmer for 15 minutes. Stir in soba noodles, cook 5 minutes more. Serve immediately.

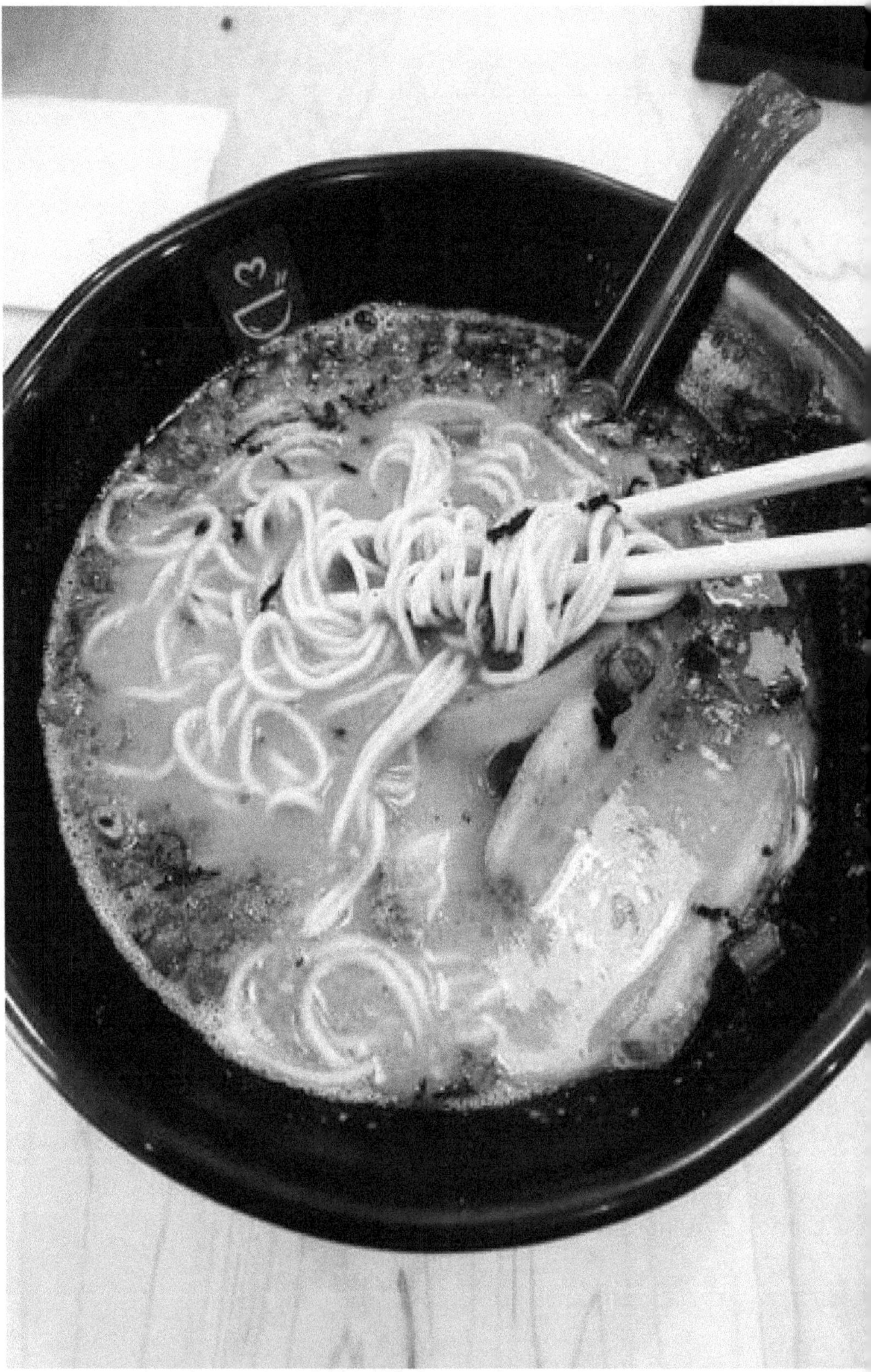

Hot Lentil Soup with Zucchini

6 Servings

Preparation Time: 30 minutes

Ingredients

- 2 tbsps Olive oil
- 1 tbsp Hot paprika
- 1 (14.5-oz) can crushed Tomatoes
- 1 cup Red lentils, rinsed
- 4 cups Vegetable broth
- 3 cups chopped Swiss chard
- 1 Onion, chopped
- 1 Zucchini, chopped
- 1 Garlic clove, minced

Directions

- Warm the oil in a pot over medium heat.
- Add in onion, zucchini, and garlic and sauté for 5 minutes until tender.
- Add in paprika, tomatoes, lentils, broth, salt, and pepper. Bring to a boil, then lower the heat and simmer for 15 minutes, stirring often.
- Add in the Swiss chard and cook for another 3-5 minutes. Serve immediately.

Coconut Artichoke Soup with Almonds

6 Servings

Preparation Time: 30 minutes

Ingredients

- 1 tbsp Olive oil
- Salt to taste
- ⅓ cup Plant butter
- ⅛ tsp ground Cayenne pepper
- 1 cup plain Coconut cream
- 1 tbsp snipped fresh Chives
- 2 tbsps sliced toasted Almonds
- 2 medium Shallots, chopped
- 2 (10-oz) packages Artichoke hearts
- 3 cups Vegetable broth
- 1 tsp fresh Lemon juice

Directions

- Warm the oil in a pot over medium heat.
- Add in shallots and sauté until softened, about 3 minutes.
- Add in artichokes, broth, lemon juice, and salt.
- Bring to a boil, lower the heat, and simmer for 10 minutes.

- Stir in butter and cayenne pepper. Transfer to a food processor and blend until purée.
- Return to the pot. Mix in the coconut cream and simmer for 5 minutes.
- Serve topped with chives and almonds.

Turnip & Rutabaga Soup

7 Servings

Preparation Time: 30 minutes

Ingredients

- 2 tbsps Olive oil
- 1 Turnip chopped
- 1 Red potato, chopped
- 5 cups Vegetable stock
- 2 tsps dried Thyme
- 1 Onion, diced
- 3 Garlic cloves, minced
- 1 Carrot, chopped
- 1 Rutabaga, chopped

Directions

- Warm the oil in a pot over medium heat.
- Add the onion and garlic and sauté for 3 minutes until translucent.
- Stir in carrot, rutabaga, turnip, potato, vegetable stock, salt, pepper, and thyme. Simmer for 10 minutes.
- In a food processor, put the soup and blend until purée. Serve warm.

Greek Salad

4 Servings

Preparation Time: 10 minutes

Ingredients

- ½ Yellow bell pepper, cut into pieces
- ½ Red onion, peeled and sliced
- ½ cup Tofu cheese, cut into squares
- 10 Kalamata olives, pitted
- ½ tbsp Red wine vinegar
- 4 tbsps Olive oil
- 2 tsps dried Oregano
- 3 Tomatoes cut into bite-size pieces
- ½ cucumber, cut into bite-size pieces

Directions

- Put the bell pepper, tomatoes, cucumber, red onion, tofu cheese, and olives into a salad bowl.

- Drizzle the red wine vinegar and olive oil over the vegetables.

- Season with salt, black pepper, and oregano, and toss the salad with two spoons.

- Share the salad into four bowls and serve immediately.

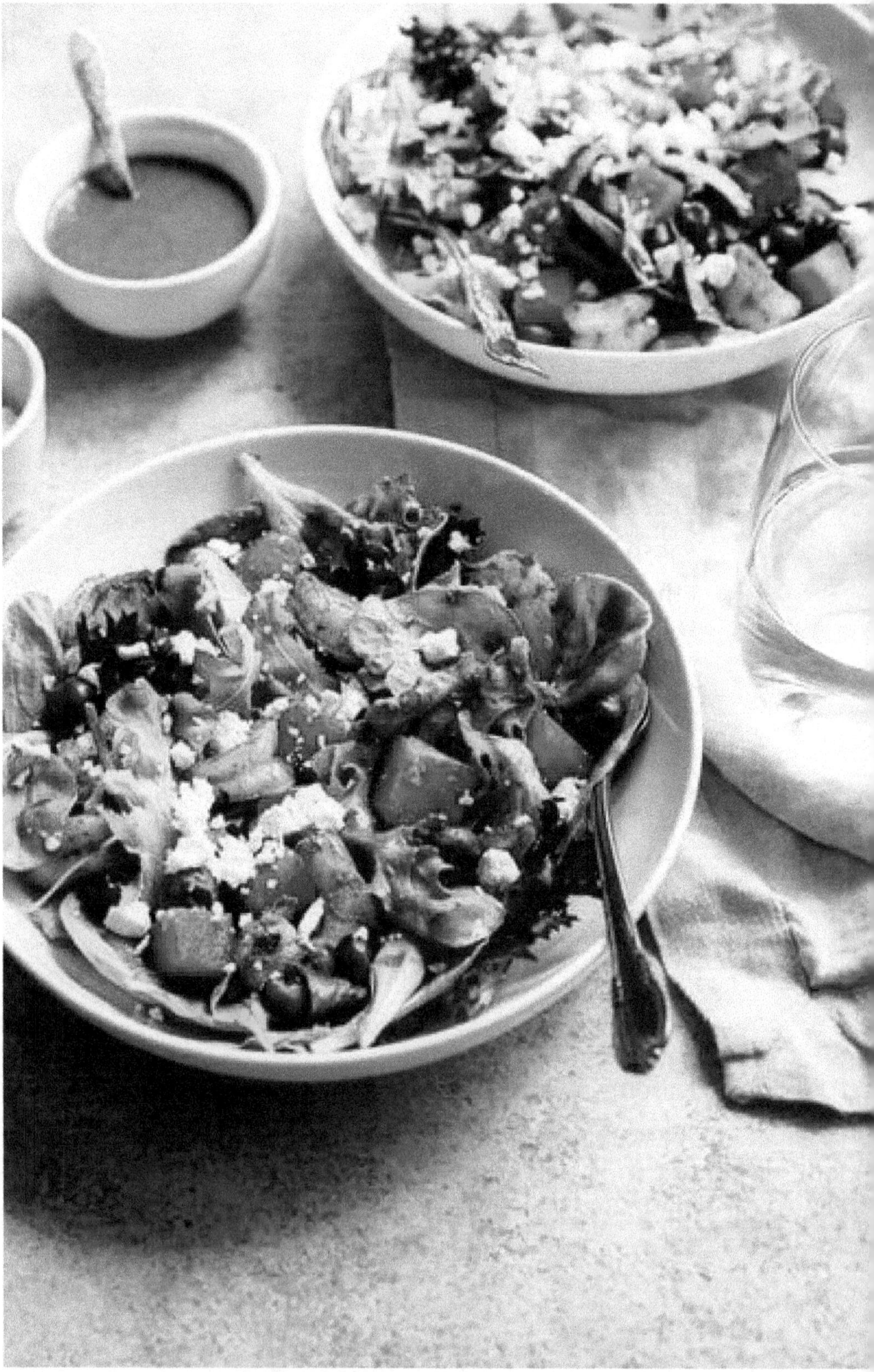

Squash Salad

6 Servings

Preparation Time: 20 minutes

Ingredients

- 2 lbs Green squash, cubed
- 3 oz Fennel, sliced
- 2 oz chopped Green onions
- 1 cup Tofu mayonnaise
- 2 tbsps fresh Chives, finely chopped
- A pinch of Mustard powder
- Chopped Dill to garnish
- 2 tbsps Plant butter
- Salt and Black pepper to taste

Directions

- Put a pan over medium heat and melt plant butter.
- Fry in squash cubes until slightly softened but not browned, about 7 minutes. Allow the squash to cool.
- In a salad bowl, mix the cooled squash, fennel slices, green onions, tofu mayonnaise, chives, and mustard powder.
- Garnish with dill and serve.

Beet Tofu Salad

6 Servings

Preparation Time: 50 minutes

Ingredients

- 8 oz Red beets
- ½ red Onion
- 1 cup Tofu mayonnaise
- 1 small Romaine lettuce, torn
- Freshly chopped Chives
- Salt and Black pepper to taste
- 2 oz Tofu, chopped into little bits
- 2 tbsps Plant butter

Directions

- Put beets in a pot, cover with water, and bring to a boil for 40 minutes.

- Melt plant butter in a non-stick pan over medium heat and fry tofu until browned.

- Set aside to cool. When the bits are ready, drain through a colander and allow cooling. Slip the skin off after and slice them.

- In a salad bowl, combine the beets, tofu, red onions, lettuce, salt, pepper, and tofu mayonnaise and mix until the vegetables are adequately coated with the mayonnaise.

- Garnish with chives and serve.

SNACKS & SIDES

Plant-Based Cheddar Cheese

8 Servings

Preparation time: 10 minutes + chilling time

Ingredients

- 2 cups raw cashew nuts
- 2 red bell peppers, chopped
- ½ cup tahini
- 2 tbsps tamarind sauce
- 2 lemons, juiced
- 4 tbsps coconut oil
- 2 tsps garlic powder
- 4 tsps onion powder
- 2 tbsps tomato paste
- 4 tsps apple cider vinegar
- 2 tbsps Dijon mustard
- ½ cup nutritional yeast
- 1 tsp smoked paprika
- 1/4 tsp cayenne pepper
- 2 tbsps xanthan gum

Directions

- Grease a round dish with cooking spray and set it aside. Pour 1 cup of water into a pot and mix in xanthan gum.
- Bring to a boil for 1 minute with continuous stirring. Pour the mixture into a food processor.

- Add in cashew nuts, red bell pepper, salt, 2/3 cup of water, tahini, tamarind sauce, lemon juice, coconut oil, garlic powder, onion powder, tomato paste, apple cider vinegar, Dijon mustard, nutritional yeast, smoked paprika, and cayenne pepper and blend the ingredients until smooth.

- Quickly pour the mixture into the round dish and spread it around well. Place in the fridge to set, 45 minutes to 1 hour.

- Remove the bowl from the fridge and invert the cheese onto a plate.

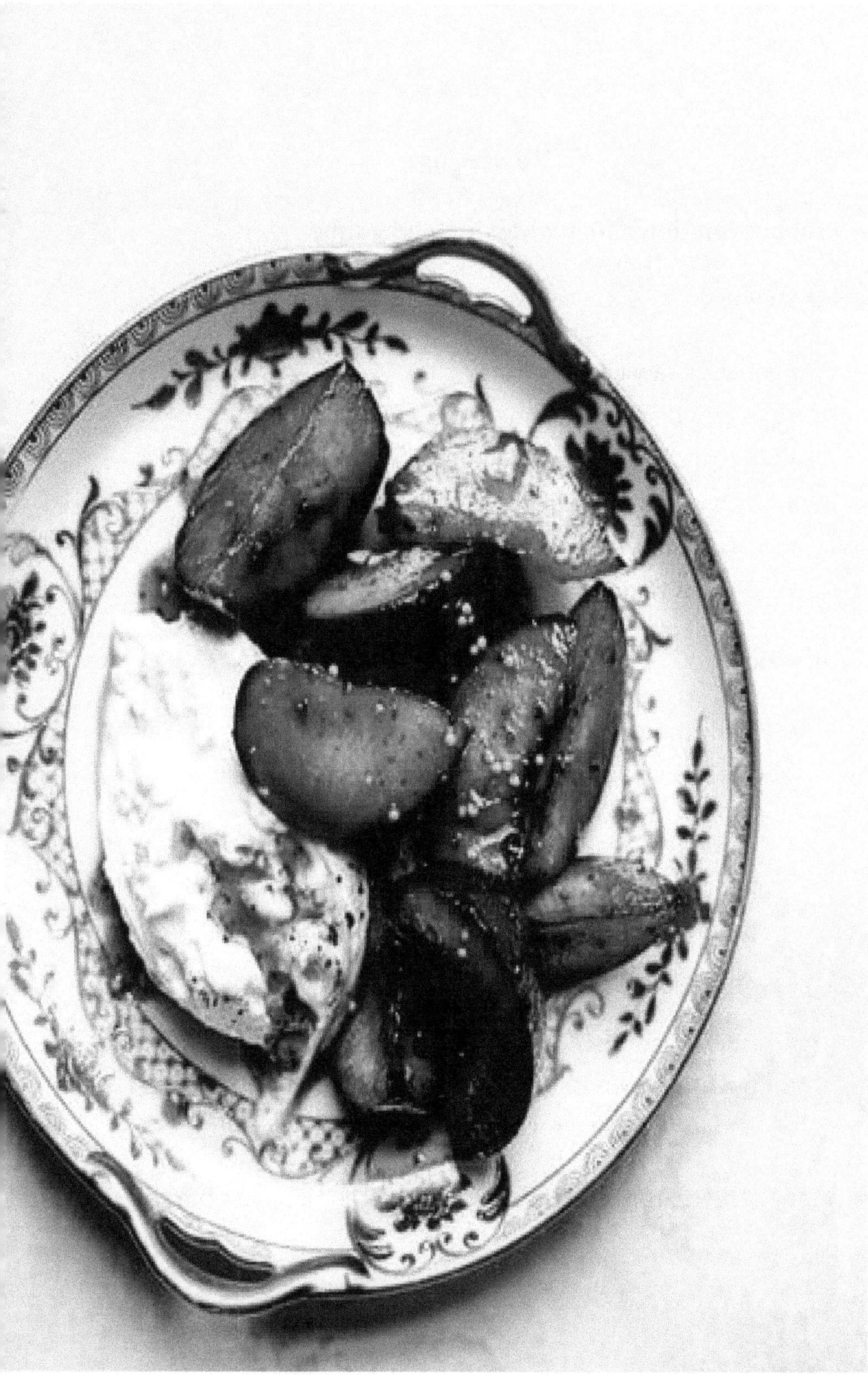

Plant-Based Mozzarella Cheese

8 Servings

Preparation time: 10 minutes + chilling time

Ingredients

- 2 cups raw cashew nuts
- ½ cup plant-based yogurt
- 3 tbsps freshly juiced lemon
- 4 tbsps nutritional yeast
- 1 cup unsweetened almond milk
- 8 tbsps tapioca starch

Directions

- Soak the cashews in hot water for 1 hour or overnight. Drain well.
- Pour the cashews into a food processor, add yogurt, lemon juice, salt, nutritional yeast, almond milk, tapioca, and process until smooth and creamy while scraping the sides into the mixture.
- Adjust the taste as needed with more salt for saltiness, nutritional yeast for cheesiness, yogurt for creaminess, and lemon juice for acidity.
- The texture should be smooth, creamy, and pourable.

- Add the mix to a medium skillet and cook over medium heat while whisking until thickened and ball-like shape forms, 4-5 minutes.
- Reduce the heat to low, then use a wooden spoon to mix the mixture until loose ball forms.
- Transfer the mixture to a small mixing bowl.
- Cover the bowl with plastic wrap, refrigerate for 1 hour, and then scoop 1 tbsp pieces and form into mozzarella-like balls.
- Use as the recipe requires.

Plant-Based Parmesan Cheese

8 Servings

Preparation time: 5 minutes

Ingredients

- 2 cups of raw cashews
- 2 tbsps Italian seasoning
- 1 cup nutritional yeast

Directions

- In a blender, pour in the cashew nuts, Italian seasoning, nutritional yeast, and salt.
- Process the ingredients until smooth. Use as the recipe requires.

Cashew Cream Cheese

8 Servings

Preparation time: 5 minutes

Ingredients

- 2 cups cashew nuts, soaked
- 1 cup water
- ½ tsp salt

Directions

- Blend the cashew nuts, water, and salt in a blender until smooth. To lighten the cream, add some water until your desired thickness is achieved.

Tofu Mayonnaise

8 Servings

Preparation time: 5 minutes

Ingredients

- 16 oz silken tofu, cubed
- 2 tsps freshly squeezed lemon juice
- 2 tsps distilled white vinegar
- 1 tsp nutritional yeast
- ½ tsp Dijon mustard
- ½ tsp pure maple syrup

Directions

- In a blender, process tofu, lemon juice, white vinegar, nutritional yeast, Dijon mustard, salt, and maple syrup until smooth.

Peppery Hummus Dip

20 Servings

Preparation time: 30 minutes

Ingredients

- 40 ounces canned or boiled chickpeas, drained
- 1/2 cup tahini
- 4 garlic cloves, minced
- 4 tablespoons lemon juice, freshly squeezed
- 1 cup chickpea liquid
- 4 red roasted peppers, seeded and sliced
- 1 teaspoon paprika
- 2 teaspoons dried basil
- Sea salt and ground black pepper, to taste
- 4 tablespoons olive oil

Directions

- Blitz all the ingredients, except for the oil, in your blender or food processor until your desired consistency is reached.
- Place in your refrigerator until ready to serve.
- Serve with toasted pita wedges or chips, if desired. Bon appétit!

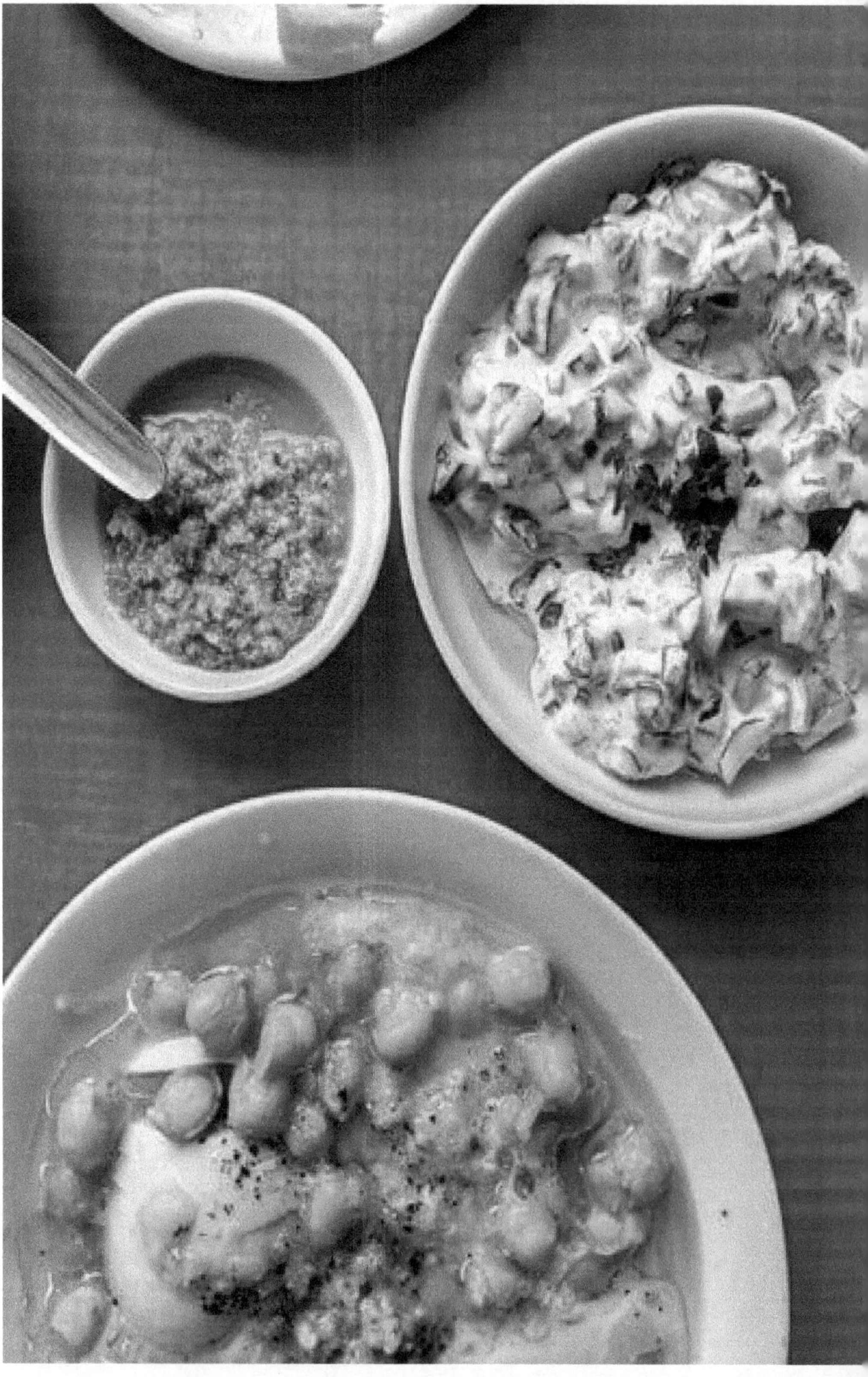

Traditional Lebanese Mutabal

12 Servings

Preparation time: 10 minutes

Ingredients

- 2 pounds eggplant
- 2 onions, chopped
- 2 tablespoons garlic paste
- 8 tablespoons tahini
- 2 tablespoons coconut oil
- 4 tablespoons lemon juice
- 1 teaspoon ground coriander
- 1/2 cup ground cloves
- 2 teaspoons red pepper flakes
- 2 teaspoons smoked peppers
- Sea salt and ground black pepper, to taste

Directions

- Roast the eggplant until the skin turns black; peel the eggplant and transfer it to the bowl of your food processor.
- Add in the remaining ingredients. Blend until everything is well incorporated.
- Serve with crostini or pita bread, if desired.

DINNER

Couscous & Lentil Curry

8 Servings

Preparation time: 20 minutes

Ingredients

- 4 tbsps olive oil
- 6 green onions, chopped
- 2 eggplants, diced
- Salt to taste
- 2-inch piece fresh ginger, minced
- 2 (15-oz) can green lentils, drained
- 2 tomatoes, chopped
- 3 cups couscous
- 5 cups boiling water
- 12 tbsps curry sauce
- Chopped cilantro

Directions

- Place the couscous in a bowl with hot water.
- Cover and let sit until the liquid absorbs.
- Warm the oil in a skillet over medium heat.
- Place in green onion, eggplant, ginger, lentils, tomato, and salt. Cook for 8-10 minutes.

- Mix the curry sauce with the vegetables. Using a fork, fluff the couscous and divide between 4 bowls.
- Top with the lentil mixture. Garnish with cilantro and serve.

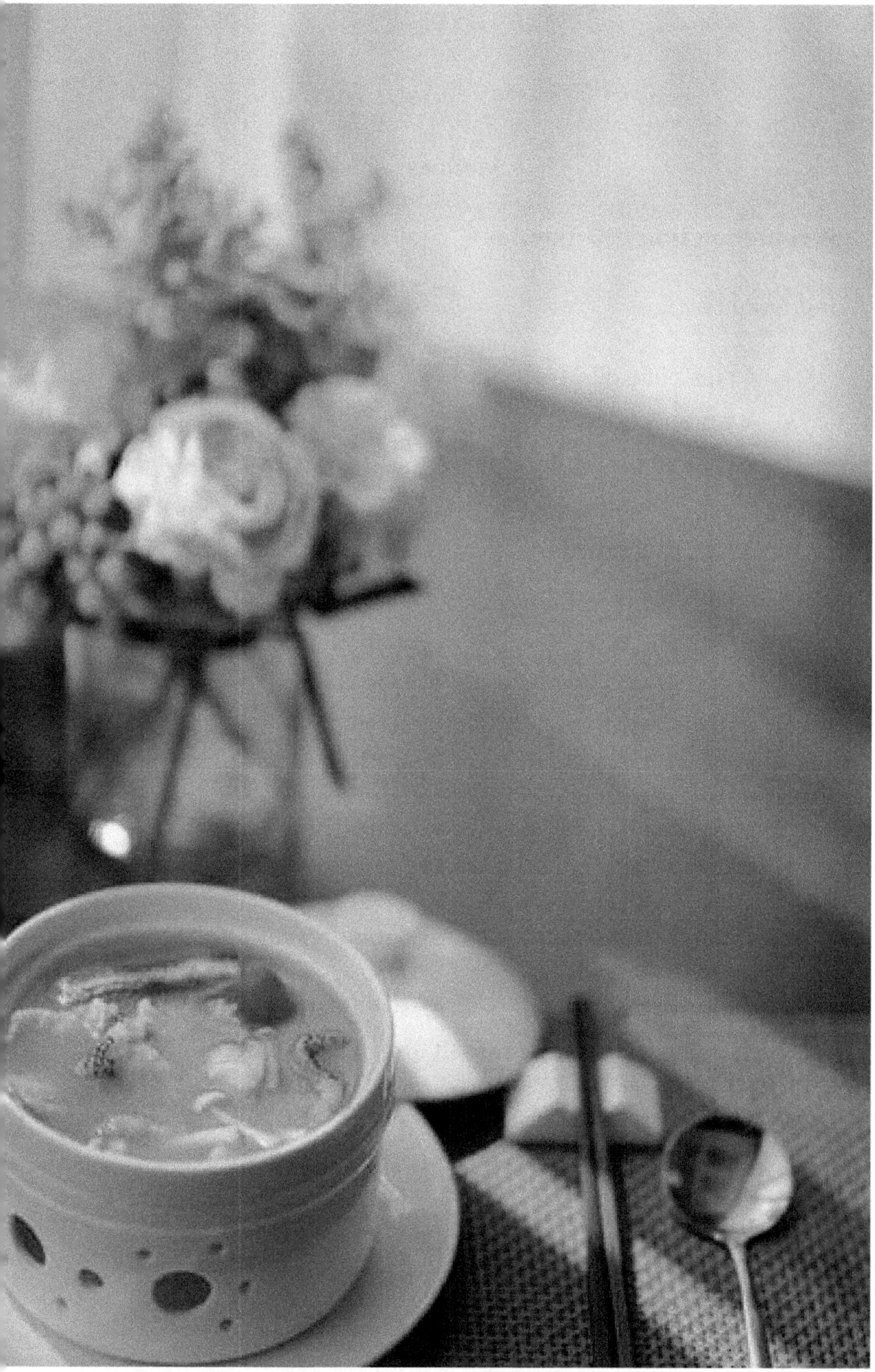

Lentil & Sweet Potato Tortillas

4 Servings

Preparation time: 20 minutes

Ingredients

- 4 tsps olive oil
- ½ onion, chopped
- 2 cooked sweet potato
- 1 cup canned lentils, drained
- 2 tsps chili powder
- 2 tsps lime juice
- 4 corn tortillas
- ½ cup grated plant-based mozzarella
- 2 tbsps cilantro, chopped for serving

Directions

- Warm the oil in a skillet over medium heat.
- Place the onion and cook for 5 minutes until softened.
- Remove to a bowl. Add in sweet potato, lentils, chili powder, lime juice, and salt and mash well.
- Divide the mixture between the tortillas, top with plant-based mozzarella cheese and fold them.
- Heat the oil in the skillet and put it in the tortillas.

- Cook for 4 minutes on both sides until golden brown.
- Cut in thirds and top with cilantro. Serve immediately.

Cayenne Kale

4 Servings

Preparation time: 20 minutes

Ingredients

- Sea salt and black pepper to taste
- 2 Bunches kale, chopped
- 3 tbsps olive oil
- 3 garlic cloves, minced
- 1 tsp cayenne pepper
- Zest of 1 lemon

Directions

- Boil 8 cups of water in a pot. Add salt and kale. Cook for 2 minutes.
- Drain and reserve. Heat the oil in a skillet over medium heat.
- Place in garlic and sauté for 30 seconds. Stir in kale, cayenne pepper, lemon zest, salt, and pepper.
- Serve right away.

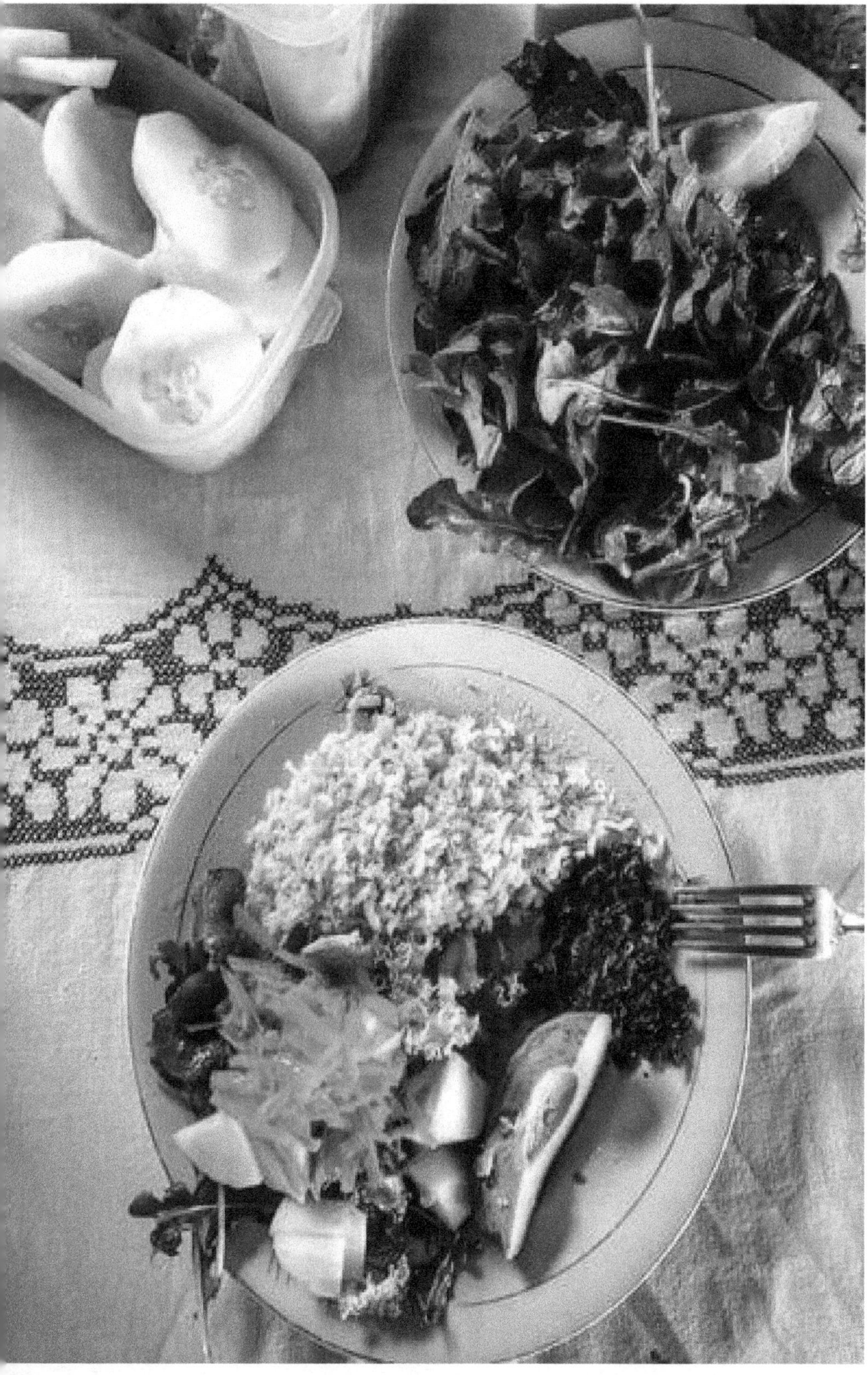

Cinnamon-Brandy Acorn Squash

8 Servings

Preparation time: 40 minutes

Ingredients

- 2 acorn squashes, sliced
- 1 cup brandy
- 2/3 cup pure date syrup
- ½ cup plant butter
- ½ tsp ground cinnamon
- Sea salt to taste

Directions

- Preheat oven to 430 F.
- Line with wax paper a baking sheet.
- Arrange the squash slices on the sheet and bake for 20 minutes.
- In the meantime, pour the brandy, date syrup, and butter in a pot over medium heat.
- Cook for 2-3 minutes. Turn the squash slices over and sprinkle the brandy mixture on top.

- Season with cinnamon and salt.
- Bake another 8-10 minutes until the squash is tender and caramelized on top.

Mustard Tofu & Cauliflower

12 Servings

Preparation time: 20 minutes

Ingredients

- 8 cups cauliflower florets
- 3 cups almond milk
- ½ cup soft tofu
- Juice of 1 lemon
- 2 tbsps English mustard
- 2 tsps onion powder
- Sea salt and black pepper to taste
- 2 tsps garlic powder
- 2 lbs whole-wheat macaroni, cooked
- Plant-based Parmesan cheese
- Chopped fresh parsley

Directions

- Steam the cauliflower for 10 minutes.
- Remove to a blender.
- Put in milk, tofu, lemon juice, mustard, onion powder, salt, garlic powder, and pepper.

- Pulse until smooth. Remove to a bowl and add in the pasta; toss to coat.
- Sprinkle with plant-based Parmesan cheese, parsley, and pepper to serve.

Eggplant with Tofu

4 Servings

Preparation time: 25 minutes

Ingredients

- ½ cup non-dairy milk
- ½ cup breadcrumbs
- 2 tbsps nutritional yeast
- Salt to taste
- 2 eggplants, sliced
- 2 tbsps olive oil
- 4 tbsps tomato sauce
- ½ cup tofu, crumbled

Directions

- Pour the milk in a bowl.
- In another bowl, mix the breadcrumbs, yeast, and salt.
- Dip the eggplant slices in the milk, then coat in the breadcrumbs.
- Remove to a plate. In a skillet over medium heat, warm the oil.
- Fry the eggplant slices for 10 minutes on both sides.
- Remove to a baking sheet.

- Top with tomato sauce and tofu.
- Place the sheet under the broiler for 6 minutes until the tofu begins to brown. Serve.

Lentil Stuffed Avocados

4 Servings

Preparation time: 10 minutes

Ingredients

- 4 avocados, halved and pitted
- 2 (15-oz) can lentils, drained
- 2 cups corn kernels
- 1 cup diced tomato
- Juice of 1 lime
- 2 tbsps maple syrup
- 2 tsps olive oil
- Sea salt and black pepper to taste
- 2 tbsps chopped fresh cilantro

Directions

- Take out the avocado flesh, leaving ½-inch of flesh in the shell.
- Place the avocado flesh in a bowl and stir the lentils, corn, tomato, lime juice, maple syrup, oil, salt, pepper, and cilantro.
- Scoop the mixture into the shells and serve immediately.

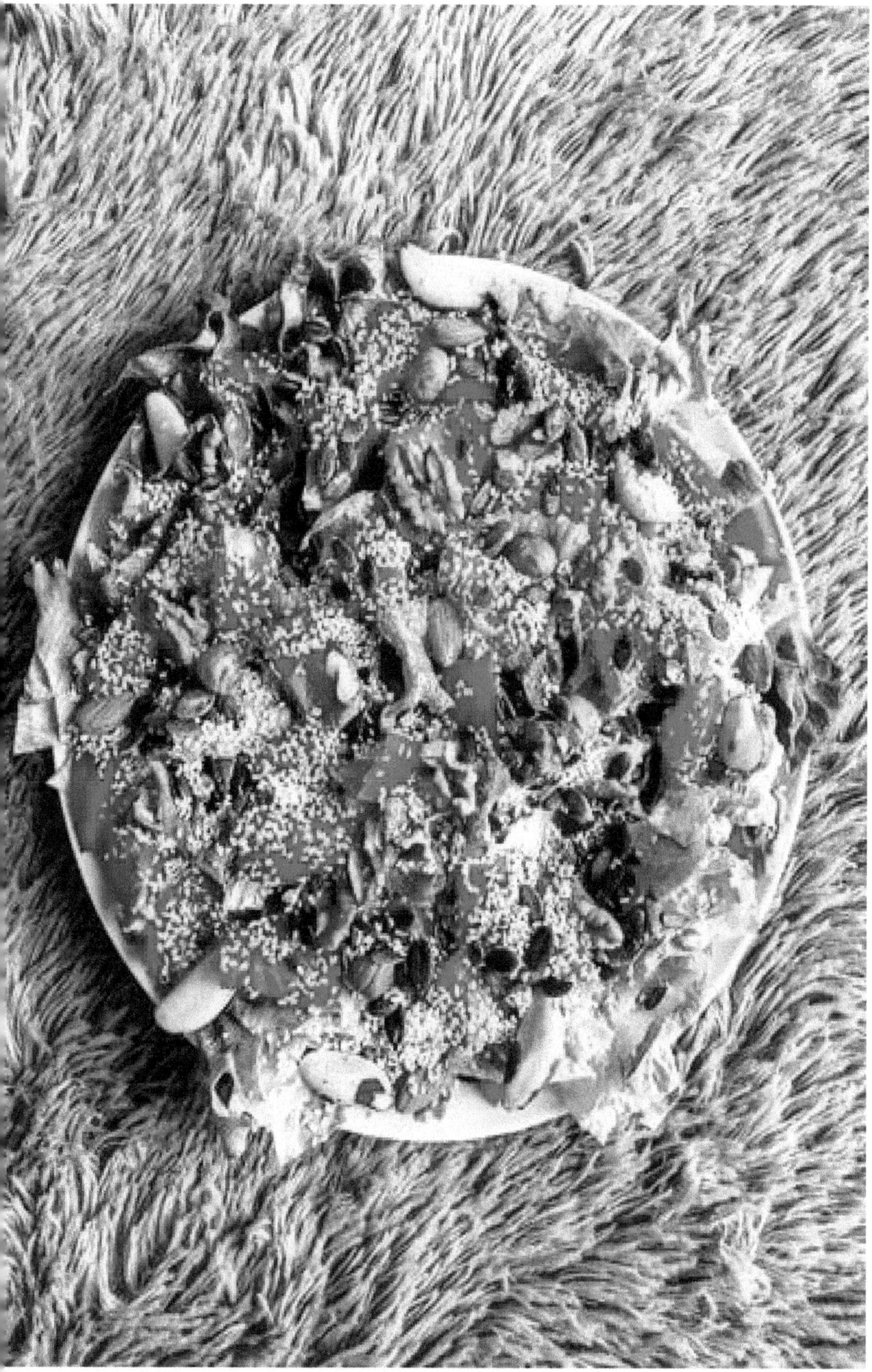

Spicy Broccoli in Pecan Pesto

8 Servings

Preparation time: 15 minutes

Ingredients

- 2 lbs broccoli florets
- 4 cups chopped fresh basil
- ½ cup olive oil
- 8 garlic cloves
- 1 cup pecans
- 2 tsps chili powder

Directions

- Place water in a pot and add the broccoli.
- Bring to a boil and steam for 5 minutes.
- In a blender, put basil, olive oil, garlic, pecans, and chili powder.
- Pulse until everything is blended. Drain the broccoli and toss in the basil sauce. Serve.

Bulgur & Bean Bowls with Tortilla Chips

8 Servings

Preparation time: 15 minutes

Ingredients

- Juice of 4 limes
- 2 tbsps olive oil
- 2 tbsps maple syrup
- 4 cups cooked bulgur
- 2 tbsps Taco seasoning
- 4 heads romaine lettuce, chopped
- 2 (15-oz) can black beans
- 2 cups cherry tomatoes, halved
- 2 cups corn kernels
- 2 avocados, peeled, pitted, and diced
- 8 scallions, thinly sliced
- 12 tortilla chips, crushed

Directions

- Mix the lime juice, olive oil, maple syrup, and salt in a bowl.
- Set aside. In a bowl, combine the bulgur and taco seasoning.
- In another bowl, mix the lettuce with the vinaigrette.

- Separate into 4 bowls and add on each bowl the bulgur, beans, tomatoes, corn, avocado, scallions, and tortilla chips. Serve.

DESSERTS

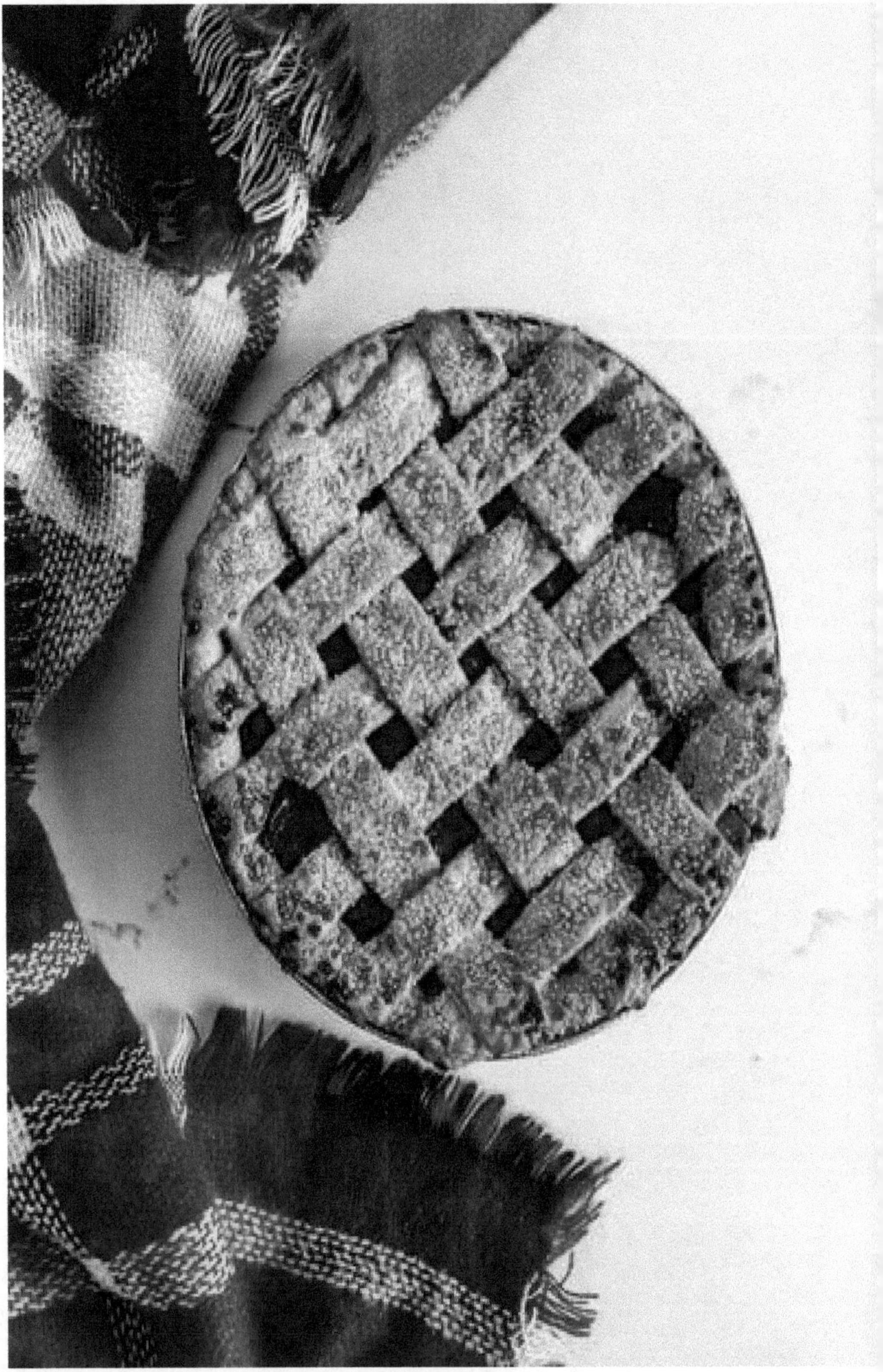

Blueberry Lime Granizado

1 Serving

Preparation Time: 15 minutes

Ingredients

- ½ cup pure date sugar
- 2 cups blueberries
- 2 tsps fresh lemon juice

Directions

- Place the sugar and ½ cup water in a pot. Cook for 3 minutes on low heat until the sugar is dissolved.

- Remove to a heatproof bowl and chill for 2 hours in the fridge. Blitz the blueberries and lemon juice in a blender until smooth. Add in cooled sugar and pulse until smooth.

- Place in an ice cream maker and follow the directions. Once ready, serve immediately or freeze another 1-2 hours for a firm texture.

Lemon Blackberry Cake

4 Servings

Preparation Time: 45 minutes

Ingredients

- 4 peaches, peeled and sliced
- 2 cups fresh blackberries
- 1 tbsp cornstarch
- ¾ cup pure date sugar
- 2 tsps fresh lemon juice
- 1 tsp ground cinnamon
- ½ cup whole-grain flour
- ½ cup old-fashioned oats
- 3 tbsps plant butter

Directions

- Preheat oven to 370 F. In a bowl, mix the peaches, blackberries, cornstarch, ¼ cup of sugar, lemon juice, and ½ tsp of cinnamon.

- Pour the batter into the pan. Set aside. In a bowl, stir the flour, oats, butter, remaining cup of sugar, and remaining cinnamon.

- Blend until crumbly. Drizzle the topping over the fruit. Bake for 30-40 minutes until browned. Serve.

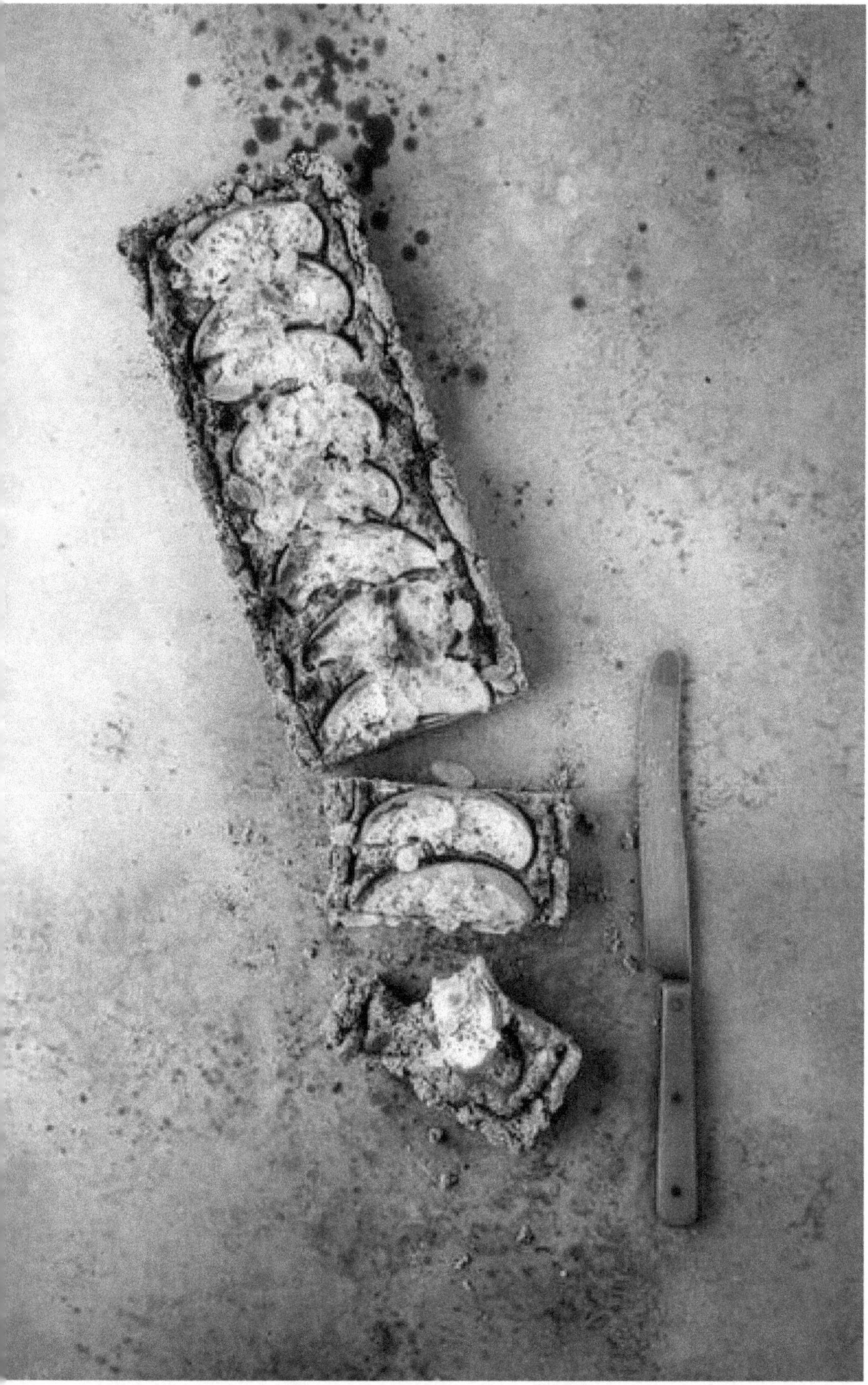

Cinnamon Tropical Cobbler

6 Servings

Preparation Time: 45 minutes

Ingredients

- 3 apples, shredded

- 2 ripe pineapples, chopped
- 2 tsps lemon juice
- ½ cup + 2 tbsps pure date sugar
- 2 tbsps cornstarch
- 1 tsp ground cinnamon
- ½ tsp ground allspice
- 1 cup whole-grain flour
- 1 ½ tsps baking powder
- ¼ tsp salt
- 2 tbsps peanut butter, softened
- ½ cup soy milk

Directions

- Preheat oven to 390 F. Arrange apples and pineapples on a greased baking pan. Drizzle with lemon juice, cornstarch, cinnamon, and allspice. In a bowl, combine flour, sugar, baking powder, and salt.

- Stir in the peanut butter with a fork until the batter resembles crumbs.
- Mix in soy milk. Spread the mixture over the fruit and bake for 30 minutes.

Pumpkin Brownie

4 Servings

Preparation Time: 20 minutes

Ingredients

- 3 oz dairy-free dark chocolate
- 1 tbsp coconut oil
- ½ cup pumpkin puree
- 2 tbsps pure date sugar
- ⅓ cup whole-wheat flour
- ½ tsp baking powder

Directions

- Microwave chocolate and coconut oil for 90 seconds.
- Mix in pumpkin purée and sugar. Stir in flour, baking powder, and a pinch of salt. Pour the batter into ramekins.
- Arrange on a baking dish and pour in 2 cups of water.
- Bake for 20 minutes at 360 F. Let cool for a few minutes. Serve topped with raspberries.

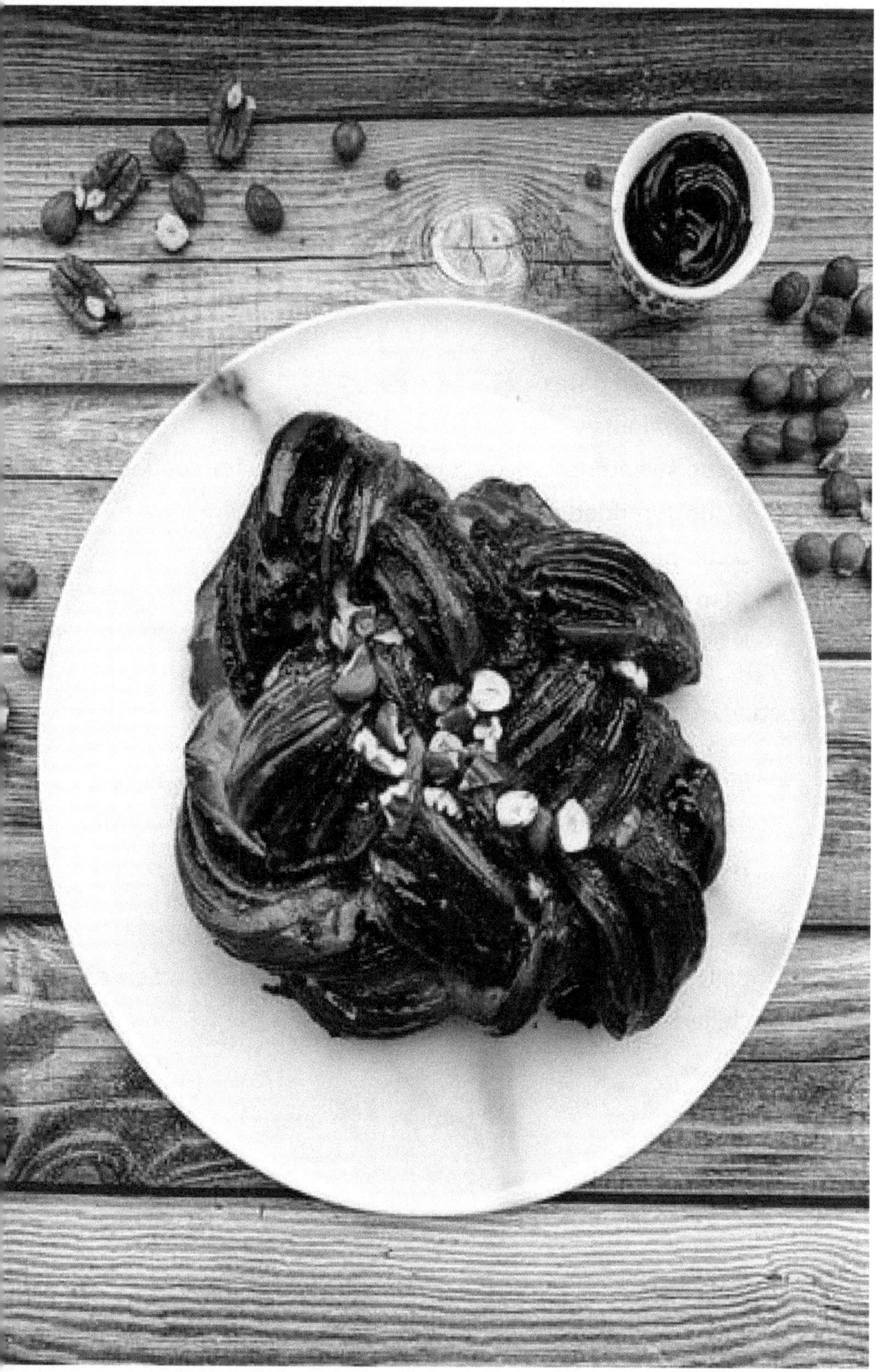

Coconut & Date Truffles with Walnuts

8 Servings

Preparation Time: 15 minutes

Ingredients

- 1 cup pitted dates
- 1 cup walnuts
- ½ cup sweetened cocoa powder, plus extra for coating
- ½ cup shredded coconut
- ¼ cup pure maple syrup
- 1 tsp vanilla extract
- ¼ tsp salt

Directions

- Blend the dates, walnuts, cocoa powder, maple syrup, vanilla extract, and salt in a food processor until smooth.

- Let chill in the fridge for 1 hour. Shape the mixture into balls and roll up the truffles in cocoa powder. Serve chilled.

Pumpkin & Mango Lemon Cake

8 Servings

Preparation Time: 30 minutes

Ingredients

- 1 ½ cups whole-grain flour
- ¾ cup pure date sugar
- ¼ cup yellow cornmeal
- 1 tsp baking soda
- ½ tsp salt
- ½ tsp baking powder
- ½ tsp ground cinnamon
- ½ tsp ground allspice
- ½ tsp ground ginger
- 1 cup pumpkin puree
- ⅓ cup canola oil
- 2 tsps grated lemon zest
- 2 tbsps water
- 1 mango, chopped

Directions

- Preheat oven to 360 F.
- In a bowl, mix flour, sugar, cornmeal, baking soda, salt, baking powder, cinnamon, allspice, and ginger.

- In another bowl, whisk pumpkin puree, oil, lemon zest, and water until blend. Add in the mango.
- Pour the flour mixture into the pumpkin mixture and toss to coat.
- Pour the batter into a greased baking pan and bake for 45-50 minutes. Let cool before slicing.

Lightning Source UK Ltd.
Milton Keynes UK
UKHW020701140521
383712UK00006B/87

9 781802 854091